Instinctive Fitness

Leaner, Stronger, Happier, Fitter!

Oliver Selway

Charlie Packer

Published by Columbus Publishing Ltd 2013
www.columbuspublishing.co.uk

ISBN 978-1-907797-26-2

A CIP record of this book is available from the British Library.

Typesetting and index by Raffaele Bolelli Gallevi

Brand and product names are trademarks or registered trademarks of their respective owners.

The information provided in this book should not be construed as personal medical advice or instruction. No action should be taken based solely on the contents of this book.
Readers should consult appropriate health professionals on any matter relating to their health and well being.

The information and opinions provided here are believed to be accurate and sound and are based on the best judgments of the authors, but readers who fail to consult appropriate health authorities assume the risk of any injuries. Neither the author nor the publisher can be held responsible or liable for any loss or claim arising from the use, or misuse, of the content of this book.

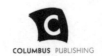

COLUMBUS PUBLISHING

For my parents

...to whom I have been even more of a burden as an adult than as a child.

Contents

Foreword

by Vic Verdier

Fleeing a used, abused and then ruined giant-sized junkyard called Planet Earth, humans now confine themselves inside a luxurious spaceship, protected from the perils of the natural environment by all that modern technology has to offer. Breathing filtered, germ-free air, they move around their ship without ever having to get up from their self-powered floating seats. They're piped an inexhaustible supply of fizzy liquid while talking to others shipmates through their own communication devices placed unavoidably in front of them. Even the person sitting right next to them is reached, not through face-to-face human interaction, but by digital communication signals. Sitting and drinking sugary chemicals all day long, their obese human bodies have become bloated and redundant, having now lost the ability to walk and move unaided.

This bleak vision of an easy but freedom-free human future was the bitter-sweet story of Wall-E dreamt up a few years ago by the ever insightful team at Pixar and Disney Productions.

What a stark contrast to the inspiring animated film, Tarzan, brought to us by the same Disney Studios just a decade earlier! Tarzan was lean and athletic, moving gracefully and powerfully through the dense, pristine African jungle - with no aids, no protection and certainly no fear. He ate, moved and lived in deep connection with the glorious environment that Mother Nature provided.

For the few hundred thousand years we've been on this planet as Homo Sapiens, our instincts always served us well, even in an environment that wasn't necessarily kind to this strange species with almost no hair and no anatomical weapon. Out of necessity, we not only learnt how to survive, but genuinely thrive by adapting our environment to our specific human needs: In the western world our daily requirements for food are now guaranteed. Our shelters are comfortable, dry and warm. We don't need to spend a lot of energy on locomotion, work or ensuring our safety. Everything around us has been designed to be easy to handle, smooth and convenient. We've even learnt how our body functions and how to fix them when they break or age.

It seems to me that Oliver Selway's explicit goal is to wake us up before we, the decedents of Tarzan, sleepwalk into the fat, featureless artificial future laid out by Wall-E. Does our future really involve us barely moving our bodies cocooned inside an ultra-protected spaceship, or are we destined to once again enjoy the natural health and freedoms Tarzan enjoyed in the past?

Right now our future hangs in the balance. Our health as a population has never been so bad and our lack of activity is creating more problems for our health and happiness than any other single factor. How could we as humans have ever become so misguided and disconnected from our true nature when - if we want to be leaner, stronger, happier, fitter - we need only understand and follow our own inbuilt instincts?

Instinctive Fitness is, in my opinion, a brand-new look at what we as humans used to do and what we used to be. With intuitive wisdom on every page, this book doesn't present a new solution to this problem so much as reminds of the solution that we had all along - had we not forgotten our origins as human animals.

Based on his personal experience and extensive research in modern scientific literature, Oliver Selway has created a program that guides us back towards our ancestral past. Using common sense, natural food and simple, efficient movements, he shows his reader how to build the foundations of a genuine programme of life transformation.

Using his experience as a Personal Trainer in the UK and taking careful note of what he has observed in his clients, Oliver has written a very sound and practical book where, aided by a great sense of humour, he shares a wealth of scientific and empirical information.

I do urge you to listen to what Oliver has to say. He explains how our instincts work and why we should never have forgotten them. It's all too easy to blindly follow the accepted mainstream opinions of scientists, experts and so-called fitness gurus. Refreshingly, Oliver claims to be none of these and instead demonstrates that our instincts and a little common sense is all what we ever need to become what nature always intended.

Enjoy the journey!

Vic Verdier, Master Instructor at MovNat – aka 'the Man in Black'

Instinctive Fitness

Background and Acknowledgements

Instinctive Fitness isn't meant as an anatomy guide or a nutritional bible, but instead as an umbrella of concepts, inspiration and ideas that actually change lives.

This is an introduction to what might be the most powerful approach to Fitness and Health *anyone* can take and, because it is intended to change lives not just add to the debate, it is written for the man or woman on the street and inevitably contains some simplifications. Hopefully, more 'sciencey' readers will understand if I have treated some subjects less than exhaustively.

Anyone can get on an aeroplane and benefit from the power of flight without having to understand aeronautical physics or how the cockpit works, and as such this isn't written like a pilot's instructional course, but rather I hope, a good guide for passengers contemplating their first flight.

I truly hope this book offers Joe Public the inspiration and motivation to stop worrying, stressing and procrastinating, and just get started getting fitter and healthier. Forget choosing between hundreds of different exercise routines or getting bogged down in the minutiae of chemical reactions that occur in the body. Just start somewhere.

If you want a book that leans more heavily on science, I would point you in the direction of Gary Taubes's work, "Good Calories, Bad Calories". It's a monumental book outlining the difficulties we face with food choices in the modern world. Or try "Why We Get Fat" by the same author, which is also top science made as simple as possible.

Having said that, if you would like to look even deeper into the truth of these radical ideas you can follow the many references provided within these pages, and delve further into the weight of scientific evidence that backs up this 'instinct driven' approach to health and fitness.

The ideas in this book do not appear in a vacuum; I am deeply indebted to the work of a number of writers and bloggers who have inspired me and have done much to popularise the Paleo movement. This is a revolutionary new way of thinking that has made serious inroads in the USA and is now gaining considerable interest here in the UK. (As usual, we are a few years behind on this side of the pond.)

In this category lies the genius **Mark Sisson** in California, who blogs harder for the Paleo community than anyone on the planet. He promotes what he calls a 'Primal' approach, but we share the same emphasis on looking at our evolutionary past and designing lifestyles that take this golden age in our history as their cue. I hope he comes across this book and that it meets with his approval. He is an inspiration.

Another figure who has helped re-launch the 'caveman' lifestyle is **Erwan Le Corre**, a Frenchman living in the USA. His emphasis on moving naturally through wild and urban environments represents the furthest and most radical application of the movement principles I employ in this book.

Authors **Robb Wolf** and **Loren Cordain** are leading lights of the Paleo dietary movement in the USA and have done much to bring approaches similar to those outlined in this book to the lives of their fellow countrymen.

I believe that the future of non-surgical spinal care and the search for natural human posture lies with the work of **Esther Gokhale**. I have used some of her ideas in my description of what people can do to escape the clutches of back pain and arthritis, and to improve their general athletic performance.

To all of the above, I often feel like I am standing on the shoulders of giants; your influence has changed the way I think about the human body forever. For that I thank you all.

Closer to home, I would like to thank **Zoë** and **Andy Harcombe** for initially giving their time and advice without expecting anything in return, and latterly for their support in making this revised second edition possible. Zoë's expertise in her field and Andy's organization has been invaluable.

And leaving the closest until last, there's **Charlie Packer,** without whom this book would not have been half what it is. He helped take my loose bag of thoughts and ideas and turn them into both a book and the start of a genuine movement. His tireless help with massaging my dry prose into something that catches the readers' imagination has brought out the full potential of the Instinctive Fitness vision. All his efforts and talents are much in evidence here.

Introduction

Despite a multi-billion pound health and fitness industry and all the wonders of modern health care, modern day humans must rank as the weakest, flabbiest, most disease-prone and stressed-out animal ever to walk the earth.

Yet this lamentable decline in society's physical wellbeing during the 21st century is an entirely preventable tragedy that could still easily be reversed.

What is 'Instinctive' Fitness?

Your body *wants* what's best for you and it *knows* what's best for you. Unfortunately decades of 'expert' advice and government mis-information have persuaded us that we *don't* know what's right for us. We've simply stopped listening to what our bodies tell us and take our advice from well-meaning outside sources who have, quite frankly, got it all wrong.

Now take a breath and imagine a leaner, stronger you – a new you brimming with energy who leaps out of bed every morning with a vigour and thirst for what the day will bring. Feeling flexible and supple with none of those annoying morning aches and pains, you smile quietly to yourself because you feel great, you look fantastic and because you're healthy, vibrant and pretty much stress-free.

Instinctive Fitness takes you back to a time before we needed 'experts' to tell us how to look after ourselves; to a time when our bodies and the environment still worked in perfect harmony and we were 'instinctively fit'.

This isn't another fitness book that burdens you with yet another set of rules

This book is more of a wakeup call that strips away the existing worn out norms and confusion, and enables you to start listening to your faithful animal instincts buried beneath all that confusing 'specialist' advice.

Peak beneath the thin facade of civilisation and the outer layer of shower gel, hairspray and trendy clothing, and you'll find a thorough bred human animal waiting to burst out. Unleashing this magnificent ancient beast does require some fundamental changes to banish those excess pounds, build a great body muscle and enjoy robust overall health, but these changes really aren't so very difficult or painful.

This is not just another fad regime that will soon pass, but an approach that works for life. Whether you are male, female, young or old, by learning how to listen to your instincts, you can build and *maintain* a striking physique and high level of fitness indefinitely. And the great news is – staying in shape doesn't involve Herculean amounts of effort or the will power of Ghandi.

By working in harmony with your instincts, not against them, staying fit becomes an effortless, enjoyable and rewarding **Lifestyle.** The Instinctive approach is simply about refusing to stress and strain over calories, 'reps' or results. It's about eating plenty of genuinely tasty, satisfying food and making exercise easier and more fun than you've ever known.

Making the decision to get started is probably the biggest barrier you face. Digesting evidence, breaking the mould and making the decision to try something new can be challenging. Yes, you're probably going to have to roll up your sleeves for the first 30 days and stick to a few simple rules, but after a few weeks of listening to your instincts you'll be looking and feeling fantastic, and you'll never want to look back.

How did we get into this sorry state?

Our modern, commercially driven world is leading our natural animal instincts astray – tempting us, teasing us, ensnaring us and ultimately betraying us with empty promises. The hard-wired animal instincts that unconsciously control so much of our behaviour have become confused. Only by understanding the nature of the modern world we live in can they, once again, be made to work for, rather than against us.

This book explains how supposedly 'cutting edge' formal exercise plans have left us bored, tired and uninspired. It also shows how the establishment's attempts to micro-manage our eating habits have contributed far more harm than good by damaging our innate sense of what's right for us. The scandalous truth is that ageing, obesity and the vast majority of modern health ailments are due to neither lack of effort nor the passing of years but to the fact we've all been brainwashed into believing things that, as Mark Twain wrote, 'just ain't so'.

It demonstrates how countless sweaty hours down the gym and tasteless, low-fat diets are burdensome or even downright dangerous. In fact, contrary to what we've been led to believe, high levels of fitness and health aren't something we must stress, strive and invariably pay hard cash for. They are available to all of us when we start choosing the right kinds of food and doing the right kinds of activity.

No matter what your age or gender, a personal transformation really is possible. We can, with the application of a little thought, reason and self-awareness, re-harness our basic human drives to once again unleash the physical grandeur that is our birthright.

Looking back at human evolutionary history, there's clear evidence that we were once far physically superior to the sorry state we find ourselves in today. Humans were once healthy, vibrant and powerful beings; we can learn so much from them in our quest to restore the splendour nature intended us to enjoy.

Today's modern world is radically different to that of our ancient ancestors – but our unchanged Stone Age genes still yearn for this long lost environment they once thrived in. This modern world is detrimental to our health in many ways; however, there is an answer screaming at us if we would just look back and learn from the past...

I foolishly failed to heed the valuable lessons taught by an experience in the wilds of Africa. For ten years I pushed them to one side until a wake-up call shook me out of my own mid-life slumber. Looking back on lessons previously overlooked, I transformed my own life, health, energy and body composition by ignoring 'conventional' advice and choosing again what had once worked so well: an evolutionarily appropriate eating style and a reliance on easy, natural exercise and activity. In other words, I learnt to treat my body in the way in which evolution has caused our bodies to expect to be treated.

With just a subtle change of attitude and a proper understanding of how your body works best, you too can free yourself from commercial exploitation and inept government interference. You can transform yourself from the inside out with an ancient, time-tested approach.

Regain control of the animal instincts that served your ancestors so well – eat like a king, play like a child and live your life to the full!

Instinctive Fitness is not another rigid prescription for health and fitness, and I'm no self-proclaimed expert (of which we have quite enough already).

Trust your own instinct. Your mistakes might as well be your own, instead of someone else's".
Billy Wilder

CHAPTER ONE

Basic Instinct

"Nothing in biology makes sense, except in the light of evolution"
Theodosius Dobzhandsky
(geneticist and evolutionary biologist)

Once upon a time, not so long ago, a man not-quite-as-young-as-he-used-to-be stepped out of his morning shower, wrapped a towel around his waist and strode confidently into the bedroom to get dressed, just as he'd always done. Nonchalantly glancing across the room, he caught a reflection in his full-length mirror that knocked him for six! Lurking where once a trim, fit and athletic man stood was an unfamiliar imposter who appeared to be none of those things.

The not-so-young man grudgingly lowered his eyes to fully take in the imposter's flabby girth, and gave his man boobs a little wobble just to confirm they weren't the relaxed muscle he'd hoped they were. He thought to himself, "I wasn't like this yesterday – was I?" This was truly shocking! How could all his frantic efforts in the gym to maintain his youthful shape be failing so badly? And why had he not noticed this before? With the weight of a dumbbell he so often worked out with in the gym, a thought slammed into his head: "If I'm like this now, what on earth will I be like when I'm sixty?!"

Never having craved the appearance of a professional bodybuilder, bulging biceps were not something he'd ever strived for, yet what stood before him was preposterous; he couldn't even recognise this skinny-fat body. (You know the look – skinny arms and shoulders accompanied by a spreading midriff).

Deep down he'd known his energy levels were no longer what they had been when he was a competitive athlete in his teens, but this over-powering feeling of deflation was something completely new. It suddenly dawned on him that even with regular exercise and a 'sensible' diet, the best years of his life were quite obviously now far behind.

However, this deflated feeling didn't last long, and his disappointment and embarrassment quickly turned into feeling of having being ripped off and short changed. Frankly, he was furious; not because he had brought this on by inactivity, eating junk food and letting himself get horribly overweight (this isn't one of those stories), but because he was fairly active and was eating what he'd been led to believe were the right things!

The hours of training he was putting in each week were obviously no longer cutting it, and were seemingly making little headway into fending off those now nicely developing 'love handles'. What was going on? He was running lots, furiously knocking out press-ups and squats while fastidiously avoiding saturated fat – all the things the 'experts' were telling him were the keys to fitness and health.

All his life he had carefully followed these 'golden rules' and the accepted wisdom that pours out from the government and media. This was wisdom he had once thought was the very reason he had always been so trim, but now it was seemingly getting him nowhere.

"This must just be the way of things," he concluded. *"Despite our best efforts, we're all doomed to that middle-aged spread"*. And as a wave of stoic defeatism rolled over him, for a moment he contemplated welcoming this decline into middle-aged, stodgy, mediocrity with an extra couple of Weetabix for breakfast.

But then a question snapped in his head, *"There must be another way to go about this; there has to be something fundamentally wrong with what we're all being told. There must be a way of getting into and maintaining a great shape without all this effort, pain and anguish."*

That man – as you might have guessed – was me.

Only two months after this sorry experience, and without committing any extra time or effort to training, I was a different man. I had found my own Holy Grail: a way to lose fat and gain muscle at the same time and left me feeling great. There was almost no supporting evidence in the mainstream media to back up the methods I used, but it was clear that my newly formulated dietary and exercise methods had resulted in the loss of all the fat I had accumulated over the last decade in just a few weeks, while developing new muscle that people quickly started noticing. What's more my energy levels were super-charged. Although I still got sleepy at bedtime, I was indefatigable for the rest of the day, from the first moment I arose from bed until it was time to sleep.

What I had been doing to keep trim clearly hadn't worked, so I had decided to forget everything I'd been told and go back to the very beginning. I thought back to 15 years before when in my 20s I'd worked closely with men who were then in their 50's and 60's. By anyone's standards they were in superb physical condition. These men were slim and strong, could walk all day and ran and jumped like trained athletes. They had never even heard of the word 'gym' or 'diet' but ate like gluttons and took the idea of 'taking it easy' very, very seriously.

I thought back to lessons I had been shown but somehow managed not to heed for over a decade and the faintest outline of an idea began to appear. I trawled the Internet for clues. I slogged through countless sites and blogs on a quest to find something that made more sense than the usual mainstream fitness advice.

I refused to believe the same worn out wrong answers that I'd been sold before, but this time I chose to do things a little differently. I didn't type into Google the usual 'get fit', 'exercise advice' etc. Oh no, for this specific quest I searched for different keywords, which included words like 'native', 'tribe' and 'hunter-gatherer'.

With an open mind, in surprisingly little time, I managed to find the Holy Grail: a way to lose fat and gain muscle at the same time.

Sure, I still didn't look like Stallone (don't think I wanted to either), but this new, fitter leaner me was about much more than just looks. Not more than three months after I began my new plan – and at 34 years old – I was fitter than I had ever been – and fitter than anyone I knew. I was even stronger, faster and more athletic than I had been at sixteen when I was a 1500m County Athletics Champion.

This isn't fanciful thinking – I proved it. To test myself, I entered the same county athletics event 18 years after I had last competed and ran four minutes 32 seconds – bettering my old personal best by a small margin. This was done on only eight weeks of my newly adopted methods of eating and training.

I now had an abundance of energy and well being that I hadn't experienced in decades. The layer of fat I'd been steadily collecting around my midriff had, as if by magic, disappeared. I started feeling 'right' in myself again and my lost confidence quickly returned. My body started feeling like mine again, rather than that awkward, strangely shaped vehicle I'd grudgingly begun accepting as mine.

Ok, so you got yourself into great shape, you might be thinking. Kind of impressive but *others have done so before – so what?*

Yes, but here's the rub:

I achieved all this without effort, extra hours training, low-calorie dieting, boring meal choices or fancy (and expensive) gym membership.

Moreover, three years on, aged 37 I have *maintained* this shape and fitness level almost effortlessly, while everybody else I saw make improvements during this time have slipped back into their previous habits and returned to their previous low levels of fitness within a matter of months. It turns out that the method I stumbled upon, besides just delivering consistent results, has an added quality that changes everything. I call it *stickability*: a quality that in all endeavours separates winners from losers.

I found out that when you make the *right changes*, you'd be able to *keep* all the progress you make. Get there the wrong way and all you'll get is a temporary fix before your body and your habits, like an elastic band, snap back to where you started.

Time for a career change

I was so excited by my new philosophy that I quit my job in journalism there and then to qualify and share my knowledge as a Personal Trainer. I was desperate to pass on this knowledge on to as many people as I could, and was over the moon when my methods worked equally well for *everyone* I worked with. Ranging from young, active sports men and women, right through to the older members of society who were starting from a much lower base level of fitness, the results were always the same: huge gains in health, fitness and vitality in an astonishingly short time.

I had known the essence of what I had just re-discovered for years, but had been foolishly ignoring it. I had previously tasted a life of both physical and mental ease in a place that was *far* from *easy*. There I had experienced the simplest and deepest of pleasures, enjoying the effect it had on both my body and soul. But naively, I believed the modern western world knew better and happiness was to be found with a good job and loads of money. Fitness and wellbeing were, I believed, just a gym membership away. I was wrong. Very wrong.

Valuable lessons missed

Back in the mid-nineties while I was still a young, skinny 'twenty-something', I spent a whole summer training to be a game ranger in the Sabi Sand Nature Reserve in the Mpumalanga province of South Africa. Sabi Sand is the birthplace of sustainable wildlife tourism, and is the oldest of all the private reserves in South Africa. It's a natural wilderness area home to a vast wildlife population, including all of Africa's top five big, scary animals.

It was here during time away from University that I spent a summer as a trainee game ranger. Family ties had led me to Africa. Learning to take groups of tourists out into the untamed wilderness, getting them close to the animals and bringing them back safe, happy with a camera full of pictures seemed like a great way of spending a few months. I learnt amongst other things how to drive a Land Rover across difficult terrain, to handle a rife correctly and how to come into close but safe contact with dangerous animals. Although great fun, these more exciting elements were not the biggest lessons that I should have learnt.

Going 'native'

Most of our days were spent doing seemingly mundane activity, covering mile after mile of savannah on foot, scrutinising the ground for tracks and scanning the bushes for flora or fauna. The plains of Africa have neither the smoothly paved nor softly furnished terrain we're used to in the developed world – but are instead a wild and unforgiving environment. The sun was relentlessly hot and the constantly moving sand caused legs and feet to tire long before they would on a uniformly paved street of a modern city. Each and every footfall was a new challenge, with each step having to be carefully calculated and judged before placing to avoid noisy, snapping sticks or hidden, venomous snakes.

Often carrying heavy weights including a rifle and provisions our intrepid group covered between seven and fifteen 'hard' miles a day.

Every so often the purpose of all our studious creeping about would materialise. On the discovery of fresh animal tracks or other signs of resent animal activity, we would double our pace fuelled with an exhilarating flood of adrenalin. We would to trot along with renewed vigour to outpace and catch up with whatever big beasty was oblivious to our presence ahead.

Our merry group of wannabe park rangers was theoretically led by John, a white Park Ranger in his early thirties. John had spent the last 17 years of his life in game parks and was clearly experienced, fit and very capable, but in reality he was not the one 'in charge'. The *real* authority was held by 'Rito', a local tribesman who had worked on the reserve his entire life. Rito must have been in his late fifties and he captivated me by his sheer strength of presence and ability to make everything, no matter how hard, look effortless.

He wasn't massively tall but stood bolt upright; he was strong, lean and powerful in a way that gave the impression of a man much bigger than his physical stature. Rito was accompanied at all times by his brother, 'Akani', who was perhaps in his late 40's, his son 'Cyril' who I would guess was in his mid-twenties/early thirties, and Akani's son, 'Roger,' who can only have been in his late teens.

Back in the UK someone of Rito's age would be accepting his advancing years, slowing down, leaving it to the youngsters, generally taking a back seat and looking forward to a retirement of allotments and crosswords. Out here on the African plains though, Rito was still very much the alpha male and very much on top of his game. He was quite obviously someone revered by the younger men in his society.

Rito wasn't one to throw his weight or authority about, so if ever there was someone energetic needed to run on ahead to check it was safe from big, bitey animals – it was Rito; if someone strong was needed to carry the heavy water – it was Rito; and if there was someone dependable you wanted at your side when it all got a bit scary, it was *definitely* Rito.

When his very much younger nephew Roger and, on occasion, even Cyril started to lose focus and flag a little from the heat, one look and word from Rito would soon straighten them right up. He seemed to drink half the amount of everyone else, seldom ate during the day (except whatever he foraged in the bush) and was always last to take his place by the fire after making sure everything was safe, secure and as it should be.

Notwithstanding the odd moments of excitement, the majority of our days were spent together, working as a team at a much more relaxed pace: walking, carrying and trotting with just the occasional sprint. Each day threw up challenges markedly different to the last. We *had* to be fully immersed into our surroundings, our senses finely tuned to both the

14

never ending search for big game *and* the very real dangers of *becoming* cat food in this truly wild environment. This unwavering focus on what was going on all around quickly became very calming and involved little *conscious* effort.

In the evenings we crept back to our tents tired but fully satisfied following a savannah scale BBQ feast. We enjoyed magnificent steaks, stews and curries of beef, lamb and chicken as well as, on occasion, more exotic fare such as impala, wildebeest and warthog. I would lie contentedly in my bunk, both hypnotised and awed by the various noises of the African night, testing my growing knowledge by identifying the local wildlife before drifting quietly off into the deepest, soundest, most restful sleep I've ever enjoyed.

Waking with the sun at six am, I was totally rejuvenated by nine or ten hours of full sleep and more than twelve hours of mellow darkness since the last night's sunset. We ventured out to greet the cold, crisp air and the aroma of hot, fresh coffee that Rito invariably had brewing. Typically we were out of camp early and completed our first local patrol and a brief morning plunge into the river before we even considered tucking into breakfast.

I felt more relaxed and more comfortable in my body than I had ever known: I held less tension in my shoulders and neck, and was standing and moving with an effortless fluidity. I realised I was feeling fitter, stronger, more alive and far more energetic than when I was a training athlete all those years before.

With my *more-is-more* philosophy I didn't consider I was doing nearly enough *hard training*, and felt that niggle of guilt that I hadn't sweated nearly enough. I feared I hadn't pushed myself to my physical limit, so would be losing my edge; but I also had to admit that I didn't care too much as it also felt that something also felt very right.

My African experience (and especially the knowledge embedded instinctively in Rito) was one I could have learnt a lot from, but filled with cocky, arrogance of youth I completely missed the majority of the lessons it should have taught me. I had, quite by accident, experienced a way of life that was very much closer to what our bodies yearn for and a way of life that we are *meant* to live. It's a lifestyle much closer to that of our ancient cousins than that of modern, sedentary man, cooped up in his stuffy office, worrying about deadlines and wondering why he or she doesn't feel fully alive or fully human.

Back to reality

Come the end of the course in September I had university to return to, so I blindly ambled back to the UK to re-join what I thought was a wiser, more 'civilised world' with all its sedentary living and regular bursts of over enthusiastic training. For a good few months I missed the 'simple' life of Africa, but was confident that, in time, the western world's 'good-life' would make Africa seem irrelevant. Sure enough, over the passing years my months in the outback faded into a fond but distant memory.

Many years later, my desperation for an answer and a new physical model brought those memories flooding back in a road-to-Damascus sort of way. The sort of health and vitality I experienced all those years ago led me to re-evaluate the experience, read thousands of articles and check out hundreds of websites until gradually I put together a truth that rocked me to my core.

The truth

It was a truth that took some digging out because it wasn't widely pub-licised, and it wasn't making national headlines – not because it wasn't right and didn't work – but because no-one was pushing it. It was a truth that didn't involve selling anything, no dietary supplements, no special exercise machines and no television series.

The penny only dropped when I started to ask the one question that no-one seems to ask – why is it necessary for humans to make an effort to get fit at all? After all, Rito and his family didn't pursue health – they *were* health, and it's not like wild animals have an exercise programme either.

It was then that I had my Eureka moment. I realised that no other an-imal or culture on this planet stresses about its fitness like we do: they don't count the calories, worry about nutrition or ask if their hips look too big. They don't have any 'experts' telling them where they're going wrong. No, they simply do what they do, and remain at peak fitness by living the lives they evolved to lead. They are naturally active, eat all the nutritious food they crave and leave plenty of time for rest and play.

I've never seen an Iguana going hard-core with weights or a Snow Leopard warming up before heading out for a 'light jog'.

I concluded that the real issue is that we westerners no longer live the lives for which our bodies evolved, and often our precious 'hard wired'

16

instincts are inadvertently driving us towards unhealthy habits of eating, moving and living for which they never intended.

Our modern world is thousands of years more advanced than our Stone Age bodies, which have remained essentially unchanged since the Paleolithic times. While we're sitting on the sofa scoffing sandwiches, our ancient body is expecting us to be out hunting and foraging, resting and playing – the only sorts of exercise we needed to take for hundreds of thousands of years.

With this insight, everything suddenly became clear to me. In order to live up to our highest potential as humans and members of the animal kingdom, we need to look back to the past – not technology – to get fit and healthy.

We shouldn't be vainly searching for something 'new' to fight heart disease, obesity and diabetes. Instead we should simply look back to where we came from to re-discover what made our ancient ancestors supremely fit, healthy and disease free.[1]

Evolution confusion

The human species came to be where it is today, not through thinking or inventing its way to the top of the food chain, but through the multi-million year process of evolution. We don't have to ascribe this rise to prominence as part of any 'grand plan' or conscious design but perhaps consider it instead the culmination of a very long series of minor anomalies multiplied and compounded over millions of years.

What follows probably isn't going to be the most exhaustive explanation of how evolution works, and more the roughest, briefest of outlines.

The basic theory of evolution is really quite simple and is made up of just three essential processes:

- *DNA is the information that makes up any living creature or plant, and from time to time the DNA of an organism randomly changes, or mutates. Any mutation changes the way the organism survives, reproduces and passes the mutation onto its offspring, either immediately or several generations down the line.*

- *The change brought about by the mutation either increases the animal's ability to survive and reproduce, or reduces the ability to survive and reproduce (or is neutral and has no effect). If the change is harmful, then it is unlikely that the animal or its offspring will survive to reproduce so the mutation dies out and goes no further. If however, the change is beneficial, then it is likely that the animal and its offspring will do better than other animals without the mutation, and so reproduce more. Through increased reproduction, the beneficial mutation spreads quickly. The process of culling off unhelpful mutations and spreading advantageous mutations is called natural selection.*

- *As mutations crop up and spread over long periods of time, they cause new species to form and split off from the rest. Over the course of many millions of years and perhaps millions of generations, the processes of mutation and natural selection created every species that we see around us in the world today, from the simplest bacteria to we humans and everything else that walks, crawls, or scurries in between.*

So in essence, seemingly minor adaptations cause every type of animal or plant to have either a statistically better or worse chance of flourishing and passing on that new characteristic to the next generation. Over the millennia these multitude of minor changes result in a steady divergence of physical characteristics between groups of animals, until what once would have been considered the very same animal had become a completely separate species. And so it was with Homo Sapiens (us).

Ancient behaviours

These evolutionary changes are not restricted to just physical adaptations visible to the naked eye; they also include human behaviours. A genetic quirk might furnish a species with more aggressive hunting skills, better adaptations to nurture their young, a taste for a new type of food, or a better defence against a predatory species – anything whatsoever that increases the group of animals chances of living long enough to produce the next generation.

So in effect, each species of animal on this planet has its own hardwired set of rules they must obey: bats wake up at dusk, spiders spin webs and bears hibernate during winter. They don't think about what they are doing – these are simply the rules they must follow no matter what.

It's so easy to see that particular animals have certain built-in responses that cause them to act predictably in a variety of circumstances.

18

Salmon will swim upstream to spawn at a precise time of the year; most animals will fight anything that threatens their offspring; a cornered animal will fight, run, or play dead; and most animals have built-in food-seeking behaviours and complex but identical courtship rituals for mating. It's almost like they are acting out a script written hundreds of thousands of years ago.

A cuckoo chick is another good example. Implanted into another bird's nest by the urges of its mother, its own instinct urges it to push rival chicks out of the nest to their death. It's in their genes. Nobody blames these animals for any of these actions – they are just playing out the instincts that nature built into them.

However, natural behaviours removed from the correct context of their natural habitat can lead the creature astray: a turkey will obediently nurtures a wooden egg, a magpie risks everything to collect shiny, man-made objects, and a domesticated dog is compelled to turn round and round to flatten non-existent grass before settling down in its blanket-covered bed.

And so it is for humans

Our own human instincts have, since the agricultural and industrial revolutions, been denied their natural environment. This leaves us with certain impulses and deep-seated desires that no longer serve us in this new, complicated, commercially-driven world.

Each individual behavioural pattern is guaranteed to have a very good reason in the wild – but let loose in an alien environment, it can become counterproductive or even self-harming.

Are we really so unlike the animals?

Humans – or so the theories go – can exercise reason, awareness and conscious control over their behaviours. Indeed, our whole system of law is built on the idea that we can be held accountable for our actions. But all too often we find ourselves acting against our best interests and the idea that we are masters of our souls, captains of our destiny and the architects of our own lives quickly starts to slip. We find ourselves taking actions that can only be explained by saying "I felt like it," no matter how little sense the action makes from an objective, long-term, self-interested perspective.

> We feel the shame of making the wrong decision, but we do it anyway, controlled by inner forces greater than our conscious, rationalising mind.

These sorts of actions, driven by basic human urges that we once depended on for survival, now cause a host of modern problems. These instincts, once finely balanced against the harsh reality of surviving an ancient world, now inadvertently wreak havoc in our everyday lives.

In his excellent book *Influence*, Robert Cialdini demonstrates over and over again that on closer inspection, man is not so very different to other animals. Under a thin layer of conscious thought lie the very same hard-wired animal instincts, which can get us into all kinds of trouble in this complicated modern world. This leaves our so-called intelligent, conscious mind the unenviable task of merely rationalising our perhaps strange, illogical actions to ourselves *after* they've played out.

Primitive behavioural drivers

It's all very well referring to 'instincts' and behaviours – but what actually *drives* animals to act in the way they do? It seems that all behaviours, whether animal or human, are driven ultimately by the essentially very simple risk/reward and carrot/stick urges, which form their motivations. We do what makes us feel good at the time. Pavlov proved many years ago in his experiments with dogs that they can be conditioned to salivate to a meaningless bell-ringing stimulus when linked in the dog's mind to a tasty reward. The physical body has its own specific tricks, signals and incentives to elicit the brain to respond with the actions it requires. Each of the signals the body sends out ultimately has both stick and carrot forms. Here are some basic examples:

Eat

Stick: Hunger pains, irritability, low energy
Carrot: The good taste of food and the satisfaction of feeling full.

Sleep

Stick: Lethargy, achiness, irritability and all the other symptoms of tiredness
Carrot: The warm, cozy feeling you get when drifting off to sleep.

Hunt

Stick: Associations with hunger feelings, itchy feet to chase prey
Carrot: The endorphins released during the 'high' of the hunt, the thrill of the kill and the satisfaction of eating and sharing with the family and tribe.

Sex

It's no coincidence that the most vital factor in a species' survival is also the most pleasurable. I'm sure I don't need to explain the ins and outs of this one…

You see, at a very fundamental level the body itself knows what it needs to survive and reproduce at any given time and provides a push to the mind to carry out the actions it thinks are in its own best interests. During the Stone Age, when our instincts were tuned to perfection, this all worked extremely well.

Unfortunately in this very confusing modern world our instincts – our well-meaning carrot and stick instructions – are no longer serving us quite as intended.

Our instincts balanced to our environment

For millions of years our natural environment threw very specific challenges at us. In order to survive, our ever-helpful instincts, chiseled by the hard-nosed rules of evolution, produced various carrot and stick stimuli to drive the correct behaviours to meet these

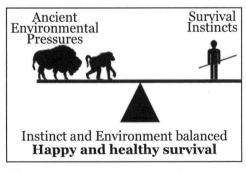

Instinct and Environment balanced
Happy and healthy survival

challenges. We are, in essence, like any other creature under certain circumstances – we react impulsively and without conscious thought. Many thousands of years ago these impulsive, instinctual actions were undoubtedly the right ones for our *natural* environment.

Our incompatible world: *Instinct versus modern living*

However, as the modern world came to be, it has grown to confuse and corrupt our deepest human instincts. We like to think of ourselves as existing on a higher plane than our animal cousins, but underneath all the trinkets of modern living, in an older, deeper part of the brain, we are still the same animal we always were, running on the exact same programming that is no longer serving us as it once did.

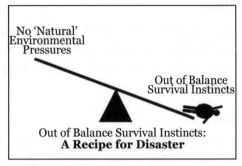

No 'Natural' Environmental Pressures

Out of Balance Survival Instincts

Out of Balance Survival Instincts:
A Recipe for Disaster

The very same instincts that kept us alive in ancient times are now being deliberately played by a modern world they simply aren't cut out to deal with.

The sorts of challenges we once faced, and evolution prepared us for, no longer exist for us. Instead, these basic drives have been hijacked by technology and commerce and are actually damaging us rather than helping us to thrive.

To find true health in the modern world we need to understand the nature of our innate human instincts forged in a Stone Age environment. We need to find ways to realign those drives with the stimulation, challenges and nutrition that our bodies evolved to thrive on.

We also need to immunise ourselves from the modern threats, lures, baits and traps waiting to hook us into the false comforts of modern living.

The ancient drives that served us so well for millions of years are not always obvious, as they've been bent out of shape and abused by modern living, but they do exist, and by becoming aware of them, you will start to respect them more, understand what they are trying to do for you, and look for ways to defend them against exploitation.

Ten basic human survival instincts

- *Rest whenever possible*

- *Eat whatever's available and tastes good*

- *Put on weight whenever possible*

- *Crave sweet foods*

- *Crave salty foods*

- *Crave fatty foods*
- *Consume whatever looks shiny, bright and healthy*
- *Sleep when it's dark*
- *Wake up when it's light*
- *Copy the postures, movement and behavior of those around us*

Because of the way technology and commerce has changed our modern, world beyond the scope that our instincts evolved for, they are constantly being tricked into leading us badly astray. We are left open to deliberate exploitation by the food industry, the drug industry, advertising, baseless nutritional theories and other forces that only have their own interests at heart. Here's where each of these instincts get hijacked.

Our instincts – *hijacked, corrupted and misaligned*

Rest whenever possible: The ancient world asked a lot from us physically, so we did only what we had to do to survive and no more. Today's world offers us few of the physical challenges of the natural environment, so we are no longer forced to raise our physical game. Our jobs, daily chores and even our leisure activities offer up little requirement to flex our muscles and tax our bodies in any way – leaving our inherent desire to rest and relax whenever possible woefully out of balance with the necessities of survival. (Perhaps the only exception to this rule is when movement or exercise is *fun* – then it can be done for its own sake.)

Eat whatever is available and tastes good: In the past, the changing seasons brought many exciting textures and flavours to our palate and served to ensure that we always benefited from a varying nutritional profile throughout the year. Today, we restrict our diet to those foods we like best and we're able to obtain our 'favourite poisons' all year round. All modern food is designed to titillate the palate in a way that over-stimulates the brain's pleasure receptors. The chemical reactions elicited in the brain set up a chemical dependency and a psychological addiction that are as difficult for some to forsake as hard drugs. This sort of food is now available 24/7 from any supermarket.

Put on weight whenever possible: Our ancient relatives' craving for calories was essential for their survival because they could never be sure when the next meal was coming along. Today – secure in the knowledge that the next meal is probably already in the fridge, the cupboard or perhaps even on its way to being delivered hot to the front door – this binge-balancing famine never comes.

Crave sweet foods: One of nature's ways of telling us something is fit for consumption is by making it sweet. This instinct encouraged us to eat fruit and honey quickly when it was available, along with any sweet tasting meat. (Many meats do taste sweet if your mind hasn't been conditioned to compare them to sugary bags of Haribo!) Today, nearly all packaged food tastes tantalizingly sweet because it's artificially enhanced with added sugars and sweeteners (not to mention the MSGs and other carefully-selected addictive substances the food industry has knowingly adopted.)

Crave salty foods: Our drive to consume food with a salty taste would have led us to consume salty meats, sea salt or shellfish – all highly beneficial foods. Our love of this taste may have evolved to guard against a lack of minerals, such as sodium, magnesium, calcium or potassium, in our diet. Nowadays, however, it drives us to consume any sort of processed garbage that's been covered in cheap salt, stripped of any naturally available minerals in the manufacturing process. Of course, no amount of fake salt will ever supply us with the minerals found in real salt, or the essential vitamins and minerals found in the meats that contain this taste, so our drive for salty foods gets stuck in an endless, addictive loop.

Crave fatty foods: Our desire to consume fatty foods makes perfect evolutionary sense. It was the quickest easiest calories available, and we evolved to use it as our main fuel when we were big game hunters on the African savannah. However, many products today contain fat mixed with sugar in a way that nature never provides. Ice cream, for example, gives us the fat we crave while simultaneously filling us with addictively high levels of sugar that damage our palate and disrupt our blood glucose levels and metabolism. The two tastes often become confused by our corrupted palate. We end up eating sugar and heavily processed carbs that quickly break down into sugar just to quench our thirst for natural, healthy fat.

Eat whatever looks shiny, bright and healthy: In nature, the brightest, shiniest and most appealing really is best. The brightest and shiniest foodstuff today however is likely to be man-made, genetically modified or artificially enhanced to fool us with its good looks. The instinct that used to guide us to the ripest fruit now drives us into the cereal aisles where the best packaging is to be found. This visual trickery is enhanced when companies spend thousands of pounds of research working out how to appeal to our subliminal instinctive urge to grab the thing with the most visual appeal.

Wake up when it's light and sleep when dark: Once, we followed the ebb and flow of the seasons, sleeping long to survive the winter and short to feast on the bounty of summer. The advent of artificial light however entices us to stay awake late into the night, allured by TV and the computer screen. We now brazenly ignore the natural rhythm of the seasons to our detriment. Where we were once relaxed, rested and alert, many of us are now buzzing and 'wired' or dead on our feet.

Copy the postures, movement and behaviour of these around us: Finally, our postures, once tall and proud, came from learning to squat, stand and move like our supreme athlete mothers and fathers – just how nature intended. Today, however, our naturally balanced bodies are contorted by modern furniture, sedentary living and the exaggerated swagger, stoop or gait of the culturally prominent stereotypes promulgated by the mass media. Back pain and limited mobility are now typical among the young and old.

In short, our animal instincts simply won't work for us while we are blindly tempted, teased and ultimately betrayed by empty modern promises of physical and nutritional nourishment.

You can perhaps now begin to recognize that the compelling instinctual urges that once served we humans so well in antiquity, are now doing us untold harm. The pursuit of an easy life and the lures created by whole industries exploit these basic human needs and urges, compelling us to compromise our looks, health and sometimes even our sanity.

A new beginning

If you're not happy with your health, your body, your weight, your eating habits and your lack of exercise – IT'S NOT YOUR FAULT! Your instincts have been led astray. Like an unsuspecting fish hooked by a lure more appealing than its natural prey, we are all falling for the artificially attractive offerings served up not for our wellbeing, but for the wellbeing of profit-driven big business.

All those unhealthy habits you could not understand (and which have not been serving you well up until this point) have simply been the folly of your best-intentioned instincts. However, once you know what's happening you can see these false idols for what they really are. You can draw a line in the sand and start again, aware of these hard-wired instincts and taking them into account to make better choices in future. Thus you can re-educate yourself against the constant traps that the modern world lays out in wait for us.

Consciously and intelligently, you can develop the ability to let your instincts work for you and not against you. The healthier your body gets, the clearer the signal it gives your brain about what you really need right now. If you are getting injuries, ailments or sickness, that's your body telling you something. Ultimately, that's what the rest of this book is about: getting back in touch with your real needs, your true instincts; the deeper, subtle shades of feeling that all too often get drowned out by the blare of commercial advertising, the artificiality of modern tastes, the desire for a quick food-fix, or the dream of a magic bullet.

Our unchangeable human instincts really can be re-harnessed to new healthy habits, based on the ways of living for which we are evolutionarily best adapted.

If the TEN BASIC HUMAN INSTINCTS ring true for you, read on and find out how you can allow them to serve you and reach a level of fitness and health you never knew possible.

Finally I'm going to introduce you to the three principles that make up the nuts and bolts of pursuing a more Instinctive Fitness (Sometimes just 'IF' from now on for convenience). You'll learn more about each as we go on. Later in the book each aspect has a dedicated chapter.

1. *Natural Movement (including natural posture)*

2. *Natural Food*

3. *Natural Living*

If you can listen to your body and make improvements in any one of these areas you're on your way to a happier, healthier life. But if you can become proficient in, or even fully master, all of these areas, the results you'll experience will surpass your highest expectations.

When you learn to listen to your instincts once again, these elements come together with a potency that changes everything. It results in a wholly new life – one that works seamlessly, feels right and provides tangible benefits that reinforce the value of these new behaviours.

The upcoming chapters will deal with each of these factors in greater depth, but before we get to those I think I need to explain why there seems to be a need for a book to tell people what 'natural' means in these contexts.

You might think *anything* that human beings do is natural because we are inescapably part of nature – and you're right. However, while some actions, movements and foods are in line with the way that our bodies and minds evolved to work best, others most definitely are not. Our environment has changed so fast that we have not evolved fast enough to keep up (for reasons we'll look at later). The story of how we departed from this time-tested blueprint for the good life is fascinating, controversial and extraordinary – as the next few chapters will reveal.

Key chapter points:

- *Follow all the rules like I used to, and you probably still won't get the body you desire.*

- *Modern humans no longer live the lives that they evolved to lead. The instincts that we relied on for millennia are now devoid of the environment that made them useful.*

- *We don't need something 'new' to fight heart disease, obesity and diabetes; we can simply look back into our past and re-discover what made our ancient ancestors supremely fit, healthy and disease free.*

- *If you're not happy with your health, your body, your weight, your eating habits or your lack of exercise – it's not your fault! Your best instincts are being hijacked by insidious commercial forces and health and fitness propaganda.*

- *We can realign our Stone Age drives with the stimulation, challenges and nutrition that our bodies evolved to thrive on.*

27

- *We also need to immunise our minds from modern industries that contrive to ensnare us in the illusion of fulfillment.*

References:

1. Eaton SB, Konner M, Shostak M (1988) "Stone agers in the fast lane: chronic degenerative diseases in evolutionary perspective." American Journal of Medicine, 84:739-749. *"Medical anthropologists have found little cancer in their studies of technologically primitive people, and paleopathologists believe that the prevalence of malignancy was low in the past, even when differences in population age structure are taken into account" (Rowling, 1961; Hildes and Schaefer, 1984; Micozzi, 1991)*

CHAPTER TWO

Truth, Falsehood and a 2.5 Million Year Experiment

"If you tell a lie big enough and keep repeating it, people will eventually come to believe it"
Joseph Goebbels
(Reich Minister of Public Enlightenment and Propaganda)

Some things in life we just have to take on faith – because, after all, life is too short. Is Andrex® really softer than other loo papers? Who knows? Who cares? However, there are other things – such as your health, your body, your wellness and ultimately your happiness – that if you choose to take on unquestioning trust could result in a life that's just too short.

The subjects covered in this book should definitely not be left to blind faith.

It's all too easy for us to believe that science now has all the answers. When you see how much we have learnt over the centuries, it's easy to conclude that we are now close to knowing most of what needs to be known. But throughout history scientists and a trusting society at large have always believed they now knew it all. At every stage of science's development the elite of the era basked in the misguided glory that 'they' were the first to really get a handle on how everything worked.

But progress and hindsight shine new light onto the sometimes funny ideas of the past, and today's scientists now look back and chuckle at the simplistic and sometimes plainly erroneous ideas their forefathers bought into. Within the last hundred years or so, some of the world's best scientists have believed the following:

- *That only a continually expanding earth can explain earthquakes and mountain ranges.*

- *That phrenology (the study of the size and shape of individuals' heads) can show their personality.*

- *That electric shock therapy and lobotomies are humane and effective treatments for depression and mental disorders.*

Ideas like this were, until recently, taken as gospel but, with this gift of hindsight, we can now clearly see just how many 19th and 20th century 'facts' were actually nothing but folly.

Even when science or new learning disproves commonly held notions, it often takes decades for the facts to permeate into the consciousness of ordinary people.

Recognise these facts?

- *Vikings wore horns on their helmets*

- *The Great Wall of China is the only man-made object that can be seen from space*

- *Bats are blind and rely on sonar*

- *Goldfish have short memories*

Even though almost anyone you ask will nod knowingly should these 'facts' be run past them, in fact not one of them is based on even the slightest whiff of proof. All the evidence suggests that all these statements are in fact totally untrue. No matter how deep a belief may have been drilled into our collective minds, the majority believing something to be true does not make it so. Anyone with any real knowledge on the subjects above probably already blushes at these spurious 'facts' being mentioned, and it'll probably be at least another 5-10 years before the media and subsequently the general public catches up.

We need to remember that many of the 'facts' we were supplied with by teachers, scientists, parents, and textbooks will be overturned in the centuries to come and looked upon as curious remnants of an ill-informed past. Many of today's truths are tomorrow's quaintly recalled superstitions.

Is it not just *possible* that in the world of nutrition, movement and health (fledgling academic subjects at best), we have got some things terribly wrong and inside out?

For me at least, entertaining that possibility has allowed me to obtain amazing results for myself and my clients that I very rarely see when 'conventional' wisdom is applied. By breaking all the 'accepted' rules I have transformed the physique and wellbeing of many, many previously skeptical people. All I urge is this:

Keep An Open Mind.

I am not asking you to trust me, nor take my word for anything, but I do urge you to look at the evidence, listen to what your instincts tell you and make up your own mind. Certainly, it would be foolish not to lend some weight to what supposedly qualified individuals say, but it's up to *you* to decide what really makes most sense.

> *"Trust your own instinct. Your mistakes might as well be your own, instead of someone else's".*
> **Billy Wilder**

This is a key aspect of what's grown to be called *'instinctive'* fitness. I am not a self-proclaimed expert (of which we have enough already) telling you that you *must* do this or *must* do that. I am not setting myself up as an all-knowing guru or pretending that I have all the answers. I'm certainly not posturing as someone who knows *all* the science. (Frankly, I would be suspicious of anyone who makes that claim.) All I can do is tell you what I do and why I do it. The results I get – both for me and my clients – speak for themselves. This whole book was written to urge you to look and listen more to your own body, to become an explorer; a pioneer in one of the last uncharted territories for many human beings: the land of self.

The title of this book urges you to recognise, honour and defend *your* instincts – your own gut feeling for what holds good and true for you. Then, by paying attention to the feedback your own body offers, you can decide for yourself whether any particular idea is worth its salt. Listening closely to this bodily feedback is essential because we are not all identical. That's why a one-size-fits-all approach will never get the best results.

If you notice, for example, that you feel tired every time you eat bananas (even though fruit is healthy and natural), then stop eating them. If you've had enough of coffee upsetting your digestion then it's got to go too. If you are exhausted when exercising five days a week, then your body is telling you you're doing too much, too hard – no matter what anybody tells you.

'Instinctive' fitness enables you to negotiate your own way through the modern maze of health and fitness, without relying too heavily on someone else's (probably biased) opinions. It's about getting to know your true self, free from any of the conditioning with which we have all been brought up.

Any logic, rhetoric or studies employed in this book really aren't another attempt to give you an alternative brainwashing. They are there simply to create enough doubt about what we're all been told – and convince you to try something different instead.

I would urge you to listen to as many sides of the argument as you can, think about the issue yourself and then reach workable conclusions that you can apply to your own life. Many of the ideas I'm going to put forward aren't just hypothetical: they are easily testable.

A little challenge to you...your first fitness experiment.

If I tell you that pushing yourself hard on the treadmill for 30 minutes four times a week isn't a good way to lose weight, then try it. Ensure you control other variables – don't suddenly start a strict starvation diet at the same time for example – and see how you fare over four weeks. If you don't get much weight loss (which is my prediction), try slowing down to a walk for 30 minutes three times a week and adding seven minutes of uphill interval sprints at the end. For best results try it in the morning without taking breakfast. See if that works. (I say it will, but what does it matter to you what I think?)

What did our ancestors do?

I'll now suggest that the above will work for you because, as humans, we evolved to do plenty of walking ('easy cardio') in a day, with maybe a little trotting and infrequent bursts of speed. We did not evolve to be regular marathon racers. The ability to cover long distances as fast as possible was not a useful function when most daily movement involved the need to quietly and surreptitiously stalk animals or forage for food with all our senses finely attuned to our environment. Crashing around at high speed would give our location away to prey and cause us to pass by any useful flora or fauna without noticing its presence.

If the above makes sense to you, I think you'll be well motivated to take this little piece of weight loss advice. If you disagree, you might dismiss it. Or you might try it anyway, just to prove I'm wrong.

> In the Middle Ages, everybody 'knew' that black cats were a source of bad luck: it was common knowledge. Your local minister would also have been able to tell you definitively that the earth was a few thousand years old and flat. What are we being misled about on health today?

Question everything ('No, why should I?')

What really matters is that you don't just take any prescriptions for health (or politics, ethics, religion, or whatever) at face value because of the perceived 'authority' of the source or because of how widely a belief is held. Remember:

The prevalence of a belief in no way indicates its validity.

Despite a tick-box education system designed to fill us with the knowledge we 'need', rather than to empower us to actually think for ourselves, there have always been people who are unafraid to challenge accepted orthodoxies. There have always been people willing to question the laziness, fear, apathy or self-interest of the majority – and it is these people who change the world.

"Thus to be independent of public opinion is the first formal condition of achieving anything great"
G.W.F. Hegel

Be one of these questioning people – a Newton, a Galileo or a Barry James Marshall – at the very least to challenge the things that really matter to you. I hope you'll agree that the longevity and quality of the rest of your life should definitely fall well and truly into that category.

New truth, new beginnings

Understanding the 10 human urges that we looked at in Chapter One is the first step to understanding how can have been misled in so many important ways. When you get reacquainted with your 10 human urges and learn to adjust for them, a great physique and explosive energy are actually much simpler to achieve than you've been led to believe. For years we've been swallowing the pack of lies that fitness and health require hardship, work and starvation. I can't think of any other area so important to all our lives, yet so swamped with pre-conceived and harmful notions – notions that actually jeopardise the dream of achieving real fitness, perfect health and the deepest sense of wellbeing.

The sad fact is that, although many people are initially prepared to pursue their personal health and fitness goals against their innate na-ture, they simply don't have the time or the will to question whether what they are being told is correct – or whether these opinions dressed up as fact might actually be doing them more harm than good.

Knowing the 10 human urges makes life simpler.

On the following page are seven of the commonest fallacies that wreck our chances of supreme energy, vitality, a great physique and endless stamina right from the outset, damaging our instinct for what is good for us.

Seven fallacies of modern fitness

1. There are no good results in dieting or exercise without serious EFFORT: "There's no gain without pain." "If it ain't hurtin', it ain't workin'". Exercise can't be enjoyable for itself – overcoming pain and discomfort is part of the process. Dieting involves sacrificing good, tasty food.

2. Exercise should leave you pretty tired because it has to be stress-ful for the body to adapt and improve.

3. Long, hard workout sessions are a great way to keep your weight down.

4. You need to diet for weight loss – eating less and avoiding fat is the best way.

5. You need to accept that you're going to start going downhill from your 20s onwards. Old age and immobility creeps up on us from early in our lives and we just have to accept it.

6. Some illnesses just HAPPEN. All you can do is eat sensibly ('a bal-anced diet'), do some moderately intense exercise three or four times a week, and hope for the best.

7. The gym is a great ally in the battle to stay in shape.

As you read on, it's going to become steadily clearer why all of these pillars of conventional wisdom are utter hogwash and are damaging you, society and the health and wealth of this country and beyond.

The aim over the coming pages is to convince you that the accepted science peddled by successive governments and the established media as a whole has been fundamentally flawed for years. When just the pure facts, without sensationalism, dogma or pre-conceived opinion, are placed under the microscope they demand we rethink the way we look at ourselves, the way we treat our bodies and the way we look at fitness and health as a whole.

Ultimately, the choice as to whether you follow the wisdom of the accepted 'experts' or opt to listen to your own instincts will impact on both your own life and the lives of any future generations for which you have responsibility. Please clear your mind of pre-conceived notions, settle down and prepare yourself for a sometimes challenging ride. It's going to be fun...

Introducing... an alternative 'truth'

For many years now we have been led to believe by big corporate beasties and the media that we are all in need of a product, a service or endless advice on how to get ourselves into tip-top form. We have stopped thinking about and, most importantly, 'feeling' what our bodies need to be fit and healthy. On top of this never-ending barrage of information on the best way to eat, drink and exercise, there is a continual stream of invasive advertising pouring into our consciousness that all contains a sub text: you need to buy or do something to be healthy and happy.

Instinctive Fitness encourages you to stop listening to what you are told and to start listening to what your body tells you; soon you'll be able to let your own inbuilt instincts for what suits *you* best lead the way.

Five truths of modern living

1. **The background noise of modern living means that nearly all of us have stopped listening to the instincts that tell us what's best for us.** We have overcomplicated a subject (Health and Fitness) that should be so simple that we do the right things without thought. We need to once again listen to these inner urges and re-align ourselves with their original intention. We

35

certainly don't need to burrow further into textbooks and magazines for answers, or indeed to surround ourselves with fancy
gyms or experts.

2. **Exercise should be a de-stressing experience, not traumatic
or involving much psychological effort.** If you are stressing
about exercise ("Am I doing in right?", "Am I doing enough?" or
if you're simply not enjoying it) then you are doing something
wrong. If you're playing with it, exploring and having fun – you're
on the right lines.

3. **Health and body composition are easily fixed when we start
eating good food.** Eating the right food starts with buying the
right food; and buying the right food means ignoring the 'bait
foods' put out to tempt us.

4. **Physical weakness and frailty comes about largely through
our own neglect and misuse of the bodies we have been giv-
en.** The 'use it or lose it' principle applies to at least 85% of our
lost physical capacity in old age, with only the remaining 15%
actually attributable to the time we have spent alive. Much pain
and discomfort simply arises through doing things our bodies
shouldn't be doing. If we stop doing these things, the pain (which
was trying to tell us something) melts away.

5. **Our genetic programming dictates that we can and should be
active, vibrant and well right up to the last days of our long,
energetic lives.** A slow, drawn-out decline is not inevitable.

How can I claim these things?

Of course any claim should be backed up with sound scientific evidence, and the good news is that we already have the clear indisputable results from an on-going experiment that has been in motion for
the last 2.5 million years – in fact the total amount of time that hominids have walked the earth. (I've also included more references to scientific papers that I think you will get through... but let me know if you
run out...)

It's now vital that we look at the results of the world's longest running,
most comprehensively researched, undisputable experiment ever undertaken; an experiment that cannot be credibly ridiculed or challenged by

any so-called 'expert' – because this experiment has been carried out by an authority higher than any modern institution: nature itself.

The 2.5 million year experiment and our supreme ancestors

What I was stunned to find out in researching my personal transformation is that our ancient 'hunter-gatherer' ancestors were not in any way lacking in health. They were in fact exceptionally strong, fit people who, assuming they successfully avoided accidents, infections and predators, lived long, active lives. I discovered a wealth of solid scientific evidence[1] that proved not only this, but also that they suffered from almost none of the modern diseases (the so-called 'diseases of civilisation') with which modern society currently wrestles.

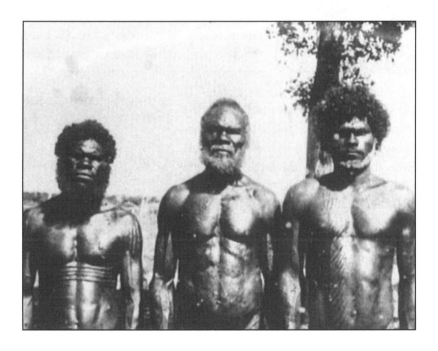

For 99% of the time this experiment has been running, humans lived nomadic lives, roaming the plains and forests, surviving on what they could hunt and forage. Contrary to the common misconception that early man lived a 'nasty, brutish and short' life (as Thomas Hobbes erroneously wrote in the 17th century), archaeological bone records demonstrate quite the opposite. Indeed, anthropologists who study the human form are united in their view that 'primitive humans' (i.e. most humans that have ever lived) were in fact strong, lean, agile and healthy creatures who often enjoyed lives as long as those we do today.[2]

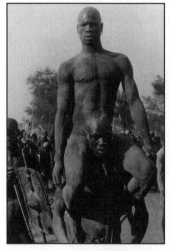

Although hunter-gatherers' *average* life expectancy was quite low in comparison to ours, this was caused mainly by a high percentage dying in childbirth, and accidents and infection – all of which seriously skew the statistics. Those that did survive these hazards frequently lived into their 70s. In some tribes it was not uncommon for there to be individuals who lived into their 90s and beyond. In other words, they had life spans that were comparable with our own.[3] And this was, of course, in the days before the NHS offered free medical care to extend people's lives well past the point that nature would otherwise let them perish.

As these early people didn't have the benefit of drugs, medical treatment or social services to sustain life, we can safely assume that they would have been reasonably active and healthy right up until their final days. In fact, only if they were active and healthy would they have stood a chance of surviving the continuously mobile nature of their nomadic lifestyles. They never had the chance to struggle on in a nursing home as older folks these days often do.

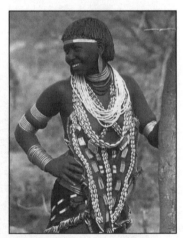

The rot sets in

However, 10,000 years ago, when the obvious allure of agriculture took over as a way of life – just a few minutes ago in evolutionary terms – records clearly show that humans quickly became shorter, weaker and frailer. They started suffering from a whole host of never before seen diseases and began living much shorter lives.

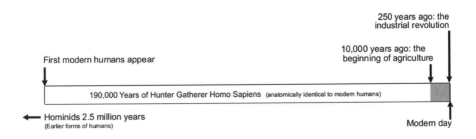

This new, modern farmer typically died in their thirties. Even the pampered Egyptian Pharaohs (who didn't personally do much farming but who lived off its bounty) fared no better. The evidence shows very clearly that the decision to remain in one place and farm the land had, for reasons we will cover later, a seriously detrimental effect on the health of our species.[4]

> If you're in doubt about any of this, be assured – this really isn't the product of fanciful thinking. Please check out the references throughout the book which link to the scientific papers that bear these facts out. See especially: "Longevity among Hunter-Gatherers: A cross-cultural examination," by Guven M., and Kaplan H. (2007).

These new agriculturally dependent humans suddenly became prone to a rash of new diseases, the likes of which still plague us today despite the advances of modern science. Of course these farmers still led pretty active lifestyles, but they did were active in the same way their nomadic forefathers were. Their life spans were also seriously compromised by the introduction of new food types made edible through the invention of new processing methods.

These food types were mainly grains such as wheat, maize and corn. With the introductions of these new 'staples' the food supply became more plentiful and dependable. With the ability, for the first time, to store excess production, the use of agriculture to sustain us expanded to a massive scale. Since it was now possible to feed people in numbers previously unthinkable, populations began to grow fast. The food stuffs the new grains replaced, of course, were meat and vegetables, which could no longer be sourced in the local area in enough quantity to provide for these fast growing numbers; so, as a species we became increasingly more dependent on the crops cultivated around us.

Modern consequences

Today, thousands of years later, following both an industrial and a technological revolution, we are chained more than ever to industrial scale farming which is producing more processed food than ever. Because of this we're now suffering from the painful fact that these foods are incompatible with good health

Moreover, not only is our food now processed on an industrial scale, but also we no longer even have to keep our bodies active. Today we can sit in office chairs, cars or train free from the need for any type of physical labour at all. Therefore, in addition to the harmful foods we shovel into our mouths, we've now added an equally harmful sedentary pattern of living. We are paying the 'double whammy' price for this easy existence every day – being perhaps the flabbiest, slowest, least healthy humans ever to have walked the earth.

We humans have still barely even started to evolve to deal with these comparatively new practices of eating and living: we make our livelihoods solely with our brains (rather than our bodies) and essentially consume nutritious-less foods made more palatable in factories. You see, when human evolution is viewed in its proper context, we are effectively still Stone Age humans, composed of Stone Age genes perfected for a Stone Age environment, and the gap between our modern lives and the life our genes evolved to deal with is filled with disease, pain, immobility and unhappiness.

It's a caveman's life

In contrast to today's lifestyle, the latest scientific evidence clearly shows that our pre-agricultural ancestors enjoyed a high level of fitness and health throughout their lives, achieved through eating the foods nature provided for them and performing the daily tasks essential for survival. However, this was far from a full-time job, and left plenty of time to fill with relaxation, play and time with their family and tribe.

So although they did have to cope with the fact that they could never take their next meal or day-to-day survival for granted, they got to lead vibrant, energetic and healthy lives, filled with plenty of time for fun, games, celebrations, storytelling and laughter. In fact they enjoyed lives that an increasing number of members of this modern stressed-out society would be truly envious of today, even if they never had the modern technology and all the apparent advantages it brings us.

More and more of this mounting evidence tells the story, not of a poor hard-done-by creature, struggling to scratch out a wretched existence, but of a healthy, intelligent and resourceful creature, living what many would consider close to an idyllic lifestyle.

'Noble savage' or captain caveman?

Why is it that we blindly accept the stereotypical image of a brutish, stupid caveman with his club, hunched stance and grunted speech, dragging his woman back to the cave by the hair?

When primitive humans first became widely known about from 18th Century fossil discoveries they were initially revered for their purity of purpose and spirit. They were seen as 'noble savages' by pioneering philosophers such as Jean-Jacques Rousseau. However, once Charles Darwin's Theory of Evolution became more accepted in late 19th century, the prudish Victorians simply couldn't accept that they could be related to such an unwashed, primitive creature.

So in their wisdom they decided instead to do what only a proper upstanding Englishman could do: deny the truth and rebrand the caveman as an utter philistine who could never be any relation to a proper gentleman – let alone their dainty but up-tight, corset-wearing queen.

Even today this thuggish stereotype perpetuates, and even your author has to resist the well-conditioned temptation to conjure up images of a stooped, grunting, bearskin-wearing oaf when the word 'caveman' is uttered.

In fact, this is just the same sort of 'rebranding' that happened to Father Christmas...
Picture Father Christmas in your head, right now. If you have in your mind's eye a tubby chap with a red suit on, with a white beard and great big sack of parcels, you're not picturing some legend handed down over centuries from generation to generation – but actually an image popularised by a culturally pervasive 1930s ad campaign by Coca Cola.

So as I have asked before in this book, and I'll surely ask again: please put your clichéd, long-held conceptions of what 'cavemen' were like to one side for the next few minutes while I re-acquaint you with our fit, agile, healthy, magnificent ancient relatives.

A day in a nomadic life

Numerous studies suggest that on average our hunter-gatherer ancestors would spend between 2 and 4 hours a day foraging or hunting for food. This would involve plenty of walking, some intermittent light trotting, jumping, bending, climbing, squatting, dragging, throwing, lifting, carrying and other basic human movements.

Inevitably, on occasion, they would have put in very short bursts of effort to sprint after their prey or to avoid becoming prey themselves. However, it was vital for their survival that they were able to recover from these efforts almost instantly to ensure they were not in a weakened state, should they be unfortunate to meet a passing sabre-toothed tiger or giant bear.

This meant that, except in occasional dire circumstance, our ancestors would never have chosen to push themselves through the pain barrier unless they had no option.

Although they knew all too well how to manage their bodies and their energy expenditure, they certainly wouldn't have consciously analysed or endlessly stressed over the best way to keep in shape. They would have achieved their supreme fitness easily and without any special method or consideration. It simply flowed out of their lifestyle; essentially a birthright, not something they needed to strive for.

Dietary choices were in fact simple. They ate whatever was available in the season. When they caught or found any edible food they ate it immediately, or carried it back to the camp to feed their tribe. Certainly (unless it can be proven otherwise) no antelope ever came with a label showing the amount of sugar, carbohydrate or saturated fat it contained. However, far from spurning the fatty cuts for the leaner meat, they would have prized and probably squabbled over animal fat when they had the opportunity. As a prime source of fuel, it would have been one of the most prized parts of the animal.

In a world without sugar, processed carbohydrates and seductive packaging, they certainly never felt the need to count calories or worry about making good dietary choices. In other words, they did the things that came naturally to them and that they needed to do to survive.

If they gave their body composition any special thought at all, their instinct would have been to try to put on weight to guard against the possibility of any future famines. The foods they ate and their active lives meant that, although they were often able to eat until they were full, putting on additional body fat was easier said than done.

Finally – and this might come as a shock to you – at a time where there was no health advice, no blood tests and certainly no fish oil capsules or beta-blockers...

...our ancient ancestors hardly suffered from any obesity, diabetes, high cholesterol, stress, high blood pressure, heart disease or any forms of cancer at all![5]

The evidence from modern 'ancient' tribes

Anthropologists are continually updating us with fresh evidence from bones and a variety of other archaeological evidence on our ancient hunter-gatherer forefathers, but this is not the only source of information that attests to how they lived their very different lives. Today there are many contemporary tribes still living on the fringes of our modern world, and although compressed into smaller and smaller spaces and continually challenged by interference from the outside world, many still live a healthy and happy existence – while all around them our so-called 'civilised world' increasingly struggles with its own, home-grown health epidemic.

Present-day hunter-gatherers like the Hiwi, Hadza, Ache and !Kung groups, with no access to modern medical care whatsoever, have plenty of members who make it well into their 80s – a feat that the UK was only able to boast long after the creation of a National Health Service.

For these tribal members, however, this is nothing special – nor has it ever been. Despite a lifelong struggle for food, shelter and clothing, many of these so-called primitive tribes enjoy great health to a ripe old age.

So would it not be safe to use these people as our guide to better health? What kind of lives could we lead if we followed their lead and merely bolstered our health with modern health care? Is it not safe to assume that our ancient ancestors enjoyed similar good health to these modern tribes? After all, they knew an unmolested, bountiful prehistoric world rich in flora and fauna. Is it not arrogant and misguided to presume that our forbearers who enjoyed a world free from pollution were either physically or mentally inferior to us? Roaming in what we today would consider unimaginable space, how pathetic would we look to them; all sickly, weak and cooped up in our polluted, carved up, fenced in modern environment?

It is my hope that you will choose to exchange an array of outworn ideas that have been holding us back for centuries with a new instinct for living that expresses the maximum potential inherent in being a human animal.

Why is 'instinctive' fitness different?

For the past 50 years, while the western world's health has rapidly declined, we have been continuously bombarded with theories and opinions about what makes us fit and healthy – but what most people don't realise (even though it's clear that we are getting steadily less healthy) is that the vast majority of the information we are given as fact is absolute bunk: useless or worse than useless.

The Instinctive Fitness model offers something genuinely new – not just a few more exercises to be repeated until bored or a restrictive Spartan diet to be followed to the letter.

You really can totally transform your body without extended efforts, low-calorie dieting, endless repetitions, boring cardio or wasted time at the gym.

What this book offers is a whole alternative lifestyle, which, although less strict and regimented than any fad diet you may have tried, does follow a few radical, but life-changing guidelines. It involves changing the way you think about key aspects of your life as a whole, and openly questions much of the perceived wisdom of our age – this isn't about training people, it's about putting them back in touch with their true physical nature.

The 'Instinctive' way isn't about placing even more burdens onto an already stressful existence, but letting fitness develop and grow naturally and organically. It's about stress-free play and eating just the best gourmet food – not enduring calorie-counted deprivation.

The key points of Instinctive Fitness

- *Superior health, not just superior fitness. Lots of programmes actually sacrifice health in a misinformed attempt to maximise short-term fitness gains.*

- *You'll eat in a totally different way to the usual faddy, restrictive plans that you've come across before. We won't even ask you to try to eat less. You'll eat like a gourmet, not a mouse.*

- *You won't need to push yourself hard to get fit. You won't be pushing any pain barriers or train like you're going for SAS selection. Boot camp is out! So are hours on a stationary bike. It won't take up hour after hour of your time every week.*

- *It's a programme that anyone can do, regardless of age, gender or how currently fit or unfit you are.*

- *It's a programme about maximising pleasure in your life, not pain. You shouldn't need the discipline of a Benedictine monk to stick with this. That's why it can be, and should be, a programme for life – not a ridiculously dishonest '3-weeks-to-a-six-pack' approach.*

Lee

Once I had proven my new formula for 'instinctive' fitness worked for me I went out to prove it would work for others. Lee, 40, was my very first personal training client to go 'instinctive' – and I assisted him to start eating and exercising more naturally through what was to become the 'Instinctive Fitness 30-Day Challenge'

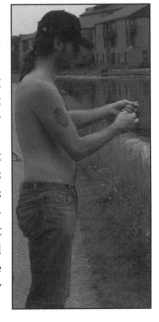

When we first met, Lee said that he couldn't understand why he wasn't feeling as great as he should; after all, he worked hard outdoors all day long as a gardener – he wasn't a typical, sedentary office worker. I pointed out that although was pretty active every day, he still got out of breath quite quickly with only a little extra exertion and that he shouldn't be totally exhausted at the end of the day.

It was sad to hear him tell me how this late afternoon energy flag left him with little interest in pursuing an active life outside his work on week days, and that he avoided anything too strenuous at the weekend in case he ran out of puff doing the day job the next week. This left Lee feeling rather trapped in a lifestyle – existing to work rather than working to enjoy life.

But the final straw came as he got increasingly embarrassed about the paunch around his midriff – to the point he no longer wanted to take his top off in the summer!

I ran him through the regime I'd been following to see what he thought, and suggested that, even though he was active in his day job, plodding away for hours in his garden work might not be giving his body the full range of stimulation it expected. I told him I believed he was suffering from low energy because of this continual slow pace. Unlike many people who, for starters, just need to get moving again, what Lee needed was a mixture of short, sharp, high-intensity movement added to his normal working routine to bring some back some of his old zap.

Lee was also eating what conventional wisdom would tell you was a reasonable diet: not too much red meat and plenty of high-energy foods, such as bread, pasta, potatoes and rice. He had been led to believe that eating lots of what are commonly accepted as 'healthy' carbs was the key to having bags of energy, so he ate more, not understanding why they were failing to provide him with the energy he needed.

I put together an exercise programme that complemented Lee's normal lifestyle and then asked him to stick to it for just 30 days.

It took a few weeks for Lee to adapt to the new style of mixed intensity exercise that I was guiding him through but, although initially skeptical, he went with it. He was also fascinated by the new way of eating I had proposed. Always strong in character, he committed to the principles right away and followed them pretty much to the letter from day one.

About two weeks into our 30-day programme, after only a handful of exercise sessions, I remember him ringing me in total amazement, flabbergasted by what was happening to his body:

"Olly, I've not lost much weight yet but – you're not going to believe this – I've had to tighten my belt by three notches!"

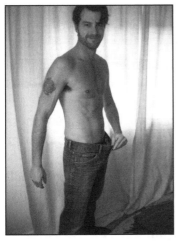

Actually, it was easy for me to believe. Lee's stomach had become swollen with the consumption of the wrong kinds of food, but when he had a break from them, the gaseous bloating started to subside immediately, leaving him three inches slimmer around the waist.

Lee saw such fantastic results during my 30 day trial he stuck with me and, just three months later, he had lost over 22lbs, could see each abdominal muscle and possessed a powerful physique that most men would kill for. But he didn't do this with masses of self-discipline and abstinence – in fact he ate like a king and he always looked forward to our workouts.

Every day he rewarded himself for his long days gardening with beautifully cooked roasts accompanied by lashings of vegetables. He always ate until 'full' (or sometimes 'stuffed'), and never deprived himself of calories. The best bit was that all his meal choices contained ingredients worthy of the very best Michelin-starred restaurants.

He says he now knows how to lose weight 'on demand' and on the odd occasion he's been lured back to the dark side on high days and holidays with family or friends, it just made him feel dreadful.

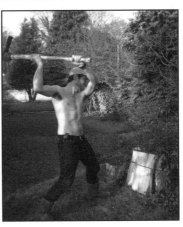

In Lee's own words:

"I still find it hard to believe a diet so widely accepted as the optimal could make me feel so bad!"

He now gets home in the evening to eat a deliciously satisfying, sizeable meal and then decides where to unleash the bountiful energy he still has at his disposal.

It might sound too good to be true, but Lee and many others are happy to contradict anyone who says fitness can't happen this way. He'll tell you how he's addicted to this new way of eating, moving and living – and how he can't ever see this changing. (Most 'dieters',

47

by contrast, are back to their old weight and old habits in a matter of months...)

I don't think you need to read too far between the lines to understand the life-changing impact the Instinctive Fitness programme had on Lee. Happily, he's not an exception to the rule. From experience, I can confidently predict that simply by sticking to the Instinctive Fitness 30-Day Challenge for a month, you too can start to achieve these same sorts of results – no matter what your current starting point, age or gender.

These methods work just as well for women, if not better. The following 'before and after' photo of Leigh, a student at Edinburgh University, shows what effect an instinctive diet and a little exercise can have. (No, I don't only train people called Lee/Leigh.)

I think you'll agree Leigh's transformation is stunning, but it's also informative. She didn't include much more exercise than daily walks to aid her transformation. I advise more exercise than this (for total, all-round fitness) but it shows how getting your diet right is the foundation for future success.

Spreading the word

Working with individuals was great, and the personal rewards were fantastic. Getting paid to keep fit while watching my clients transform in front of my very eyes was a buzz, but I soon realised that I was only going to have an impact on a very few people, and something more ambitious was needed if I was to spread the word wider. A new 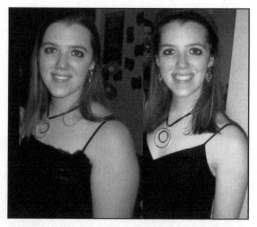 approach was required if I was to pass this precious hidden knowledge on to everyone who desperately needed it.

Nowadays, through the Instinctive Fitness Programme I have the privilege to have a radical impact on people's lives, transforming their physiques, health, wellbeing, and athletic potential. I raise awareness of the truth behind the lies we've been sold, helping people everywhere to start tapping into the power of our lost ancestry with the ever-popular 30-day transformation package that can be found at www.instinctive-fitness.com.

At Instinctive Fitness we gather the combined wisdom from many expert sources to provide a one-stop resource to start living a life that honours the instincts and inheritance of the natural health we all already possess. It provides not just advice and ideas to help people rediscover their entitlement to be fit and healthy but, most importantly, offers a completely new mental approach to health and fitness.

We remove the burden of forced exercise and restricted diets, and go back to using our bodies as they were intended: eating, sleeping and playing without target weights or performance goals, and certainly without added pressure or guilt.

All things considered...

It's shameful the way 'big business' advertising via the media has led us all to believe our health and physical prowess is beyond our control. Advertising, TV and propaganda often implies we are in some way 'broken' or in need of fixing. As a society we've been left feeling confused, paranoid and desperately looking outside ourselves for new answers. We naively listen to anyone who shouts loudly enough offering us the latest new wonder product/diet or super supplement.

We have been conditioned to consider ourselves weak, flawed and in need of some kind of outside assistance, but I aim to prove to you that every one of us has far more potential than we may ever dare dream. I promise to re-introduce you to the real truth if you can suspend your current beliefs and look once again at your body through the indisputably wise eyes of your ancestors.

But please, as previously said, don't accept the ideas offer in this book blindly; question them, think about them – but ultimately allow your *gut instinct* to tell you whether your ancestors were right all along. These ideas and concepts may inspire you or they may invoke a hostile reaction – but ultimately the choice is yours whether you choose to give them a try for yourself. If you don't give it a go, it really doesn't matter what you think of the theory, as you'll never *know* how it could work for you.

Are you ready to hear an alternative truth: an ancient truth that tells us fitness does come naturally? A truth that enables health and wellness to blossom without effort or stress?

'Instinctive' fitness means you no longer need listen to all those experts who'd have you believe you're not in control of your body. You'll no longer need to heed the wisdom that convinces you that you're powerless. This is an opportunity for you to retake command and mastership of your body and mind to unleash your magnificent 'caveperson' within!

Key chapter points:

This chapter has made the case that we should realign ourselves with the powerful instincts nature provided for us with a new vision, logical thinking, and some new habits. We can get back on our evolutionary path, the true road to becoming our best possible selves.

- *Don't believe something just because it's commonly accepted. The health and fitness industry is founded on seven wasteful, sometimes damaging fallacies.*

- *Our knowledge of human evolution is the perfect guide to staying fit and well, as this experiment has been running for 2.5 million years.*

- *After 10,000 years, humans have still not evolved to new practices such as making a living solely with our brains and eating heavily-processed foods.*

- *If we learn to appreciate the bare facts of our evolutionary past and the reason for our evolutionary drives, we can restore an instinct for optimum performance and healthful living that has been lost through insidiously harmful modern trends.*

References:

1. Dunn FL (1968) "Epidemiological factors: health and disease in hunter-gatherers." In: Man the Hunter, eds. Lee RB, DeVore I; Aldine Publishing, Chicago, pp. 221-228.

2. Guven M, Kaplan H (2007) "Longevity among Hunter-Gatherers: A cross cultural examination." [Online] Available at: http://www.anth.ucsb.edu/faculty/gurven/papers/pdrdraft04182006.pdf

3. Ho K-J et al. (1971) "Studies on the Masai." Archeological Pathology, 91:387; Mann GV, et al. (1972) "Atherosclerosis in the Maasai." American Journal of Epidemiology, 95:26-37

4. Dr. Richard G. Cutler, molecular gerontologist and longevity expert from the US National Institute for Ageing, estimates that, based on laboratory analysis of skeletal remains, the "maximum lifespan potential" of Homo Sapiens of 15,000 years ago was 91 years of age.

5. Carerra-Bastos P, Fontes-Villalba M, O'Keefe JH et al. (2011) "The western diet and lifestyle and diseases of civilization" [Online] Available at: http://dx.doi.org/10.2147/RRCC.S16919, 15-35

CHAPTER THREE

From Bad to Worse

"It isn't that they can't see the solution. It is that they can't even see the problem"
G.K. Chesterton

In this short chapter I'm going to briefly sum up the current situation with regard to the UK's health. If you're anywhere else in the western world reading this, the story is pretty much the same and just as painful to read.

If you're ready to give the background info a miss and go directly to the practical details, then skip straight to Chapter six where we look first at exercise – or what we prefer to call *Natural Movement*. If however, you want the complete picture and the full motivation to push through with the master plan, I recommend you sit tight for another couple of chapters so you can see how the *whole* jigsaw fits together.

Is the NHS getting it wrong?

Medical care has continued to improve in all kinds of ways over recent decades and many diseases that might have killed us thirty years ago can now be easily cured with new treatments. This can only be good, but it does reflect a continued bias of the medical community towards treating diseases rather than preventing them in the first place.

Only with an emphasis on long-term, on-going measures to prevent physical decline, promote health and stave off disease – rather than just problem fixing – will we be able to prevent expensive future medical intervention being required so frequently and increase the quality of life for a whole nation.

The medical establishment has, in my opinion, been too focused from day one on treating symptoms rather than looking for and heading off the underlying causes of poor health.

51

Thomas Edison (1847 – 1931, who held the patent for the first incandescent light) has not yet been proved right when he said: "The doctor of the future will give no medicine, but will interest her or his patients in the care of the human frame, in a proper diet, and in the cause and prevention of disease".

Although we are becoming better than ever at relieving nasty symptoms once individuals develop health problems, it has to be acknowledged that in the modern western world disease is rampant.

Here are a few bald statistics:[1]

- *One in two men will be diagnosed with cancer at some point in their lives (with the figure for women not much better)*

- *As many as one in three deaths this year will be from heart disease.*

- *7 out of 10 adults have high blood pressure. Even half of under 35s have an unhealthy level, (according to a report by Lloyd's Pharmacy in Feb 2012)*

- *Obesity, which is the fifth leading risk factor for global deaths, is a growing problem (no pun intended) and has doubled across the world since 1980. Additionally, almost one in four adults in England was classified as obese in 2009. 44% of men and 33% of women were classified as overweight in the same year*

- *The obesity situation for children is even more worrying. Despite their youth, 3 in 10 children under 15 were also classified as overweight or obese in 2009. In the same year, only one in five children were found to be eating five portions of vegetables a day*

- *For adults and children an increased BMI (Body Mass Index) is associated with:*

  - *cardiovascular diseases (mainly heart disease and stroke, the leading cause of death in 2009)*

  - *diabetes*

  - *musculoskeletal disorders (especially osteoarthritis – a highly disabling degenerative disease of the joints)*

  - *some cancers (especially endometrial, breast, and colon)*

In short: if you are carrying too much body fat, take your head out of the sand and act now!

It's all a big fat lie

If most people were asked "what's causing our very modern obesity epidemic"? They'd more than likely confidently chirp up: "Too much fat!"

And they could be forgiven for thinking this because almost *everyone* believes fat makes you fat: the doctors tell you so, the media tell you so, and the 'health food' movement certainly tells you so. But it's this very widely prevalent belief that is feeding a population struggling and failing to lose weight and remain healthy. You see, the whole time we've been concerning ourselves with all the 'naughty fats', the real culprit – the one causing our waistlines to expand, and our health to falter – has been creeping up on us while we're looking the other way.

It's not about avoiding fat!

We have to accept it: **we have been given the wrong advice on fat**. The prescription we have been given for a trim figure and a healthy heart is wrong. It's been tried, tested and found wanting.

It's simply __not__ an excess of saturated fat making us, as a nation, horribly overweight.

There are, especially among intelligent, thinking groups of people, very few individuals who are overweight because they consume too many of their calories in the form of fat. They generally avoid it as much as they can, just as they're been taught. Perhaps the only people who don't are those who eat at burger-bar type restaurants like McDonald's on a more than daily basis.... and that's not you, is it? In fact, that's not most people.

McDonald's, although not a restaurant I'd recommend, makes for an instructive example. If we analyse a 'fat-drenched', Happy Meal® we find that's it's not really the fat that's driving the problem. In this lovely little combo (cheese burger, large fries and a milk shake) there are 42 grams of fat (which isn't a small amount) *but there are 109 grams of carbohydrate* (contained mainly in the fries and the bun.)*

---

* Yes, I am aware that there are four calories in every gram of carbohydrate and nine calories in every gram of fat but, if you work it out, there are still more calories coming from the bun and chips.

I choose to look at McDonald's meals, not because I suspect you are a secret junk-food addict, but because I hope you can see that, even using this extreme, fat-heavy example, the carbs are feeding the problem at least as much as the fat.

As much as it's healthy to avoid some particular types of dangerous fat, the unavoidable fact is that it's the consumption of processed, energy-dense, nutrient-light *carbohydrate* that is driving the obesity epidemic.

The figures bear this out. During 2008/09, **the UK population was eating less saturated fat than at any point in the past**[1]. In fact we've generally been obediently doing what we've been told for decades. We were informed that we got fat and prone to heart disease because we ate too much fat – so we largely stopped eating it. As a result of this, a perfectly natural, healthy source of energy and good health has been vilified in the national consciousness for the last half century.

(Admittedly the 'fat makes you fat' claim has an innate sense of intuitive logic to it, but that doesn't make it true – just easy to believe.)

The point that simply cannot be avoided any longer is that, despite our general compliance with the government's 'low-fat' health advice, obesity shows no signs of doing anything other than becoming *more* common.

I beg you to suspend everything you've been told up to now, and look at the evidence...

The Inuits

For thousands of years the native population of what is now called Alaska lived on a diet consisting almost entirely of animal fat. For generations they consumed the fat of seals and walruses but suffered from absolutely no heart disease, no diabetes and no obesity. In the latter part of the last century with new communication channels and trade coming into their remote homeland, they have adopted western ideologies and new products into their lifestyles.

Over this period a new generation has grown up ever more reliant on carbohydrate-rich foods containing wheat and sugar, and the Inuit now find themselves joining in the sad decline that the UK and much of the rest of the western world has experienced.

Even though the UK's total calorific intake has fallen since 1974, its consumption of complex carbohydrates in the form of bread, potatoes, rice, pasta, etc. has grown hand in hand with its collective waistline. Our increasing dependence on starchy, carbohydrate-filled food to feed our fast food lifestyles in preference to healthy meats and vegetables is strong evidence for the fact that focusing our attention on lowering the consumption of fat in order to eat fewer calories does not lead to sustained body fat loss.

Perversely, our modern thinking on food has created another side to the obesity coin. Anorexia is a serious mind disorder manifesting itself in abnormally low calorie intake and subsequent malnutrition. Our obsession with diet, exercise and body shape is breeding an unhealthy attitude to eating and a misjudged emphasis on thinness over health. Those touting the blinkered low-fat/low-calorie message have to look at the evidence before their eyes and take responsibility for its dangerous extremes.

Get up and move!

Another issue the western world faces is that of immobility. With an ageing population, the number of people who lose their mobility only continues to grow. Lack of mobility is not only a massive problem for those who suffer from not being able to get about – doing chores, the shopping, socialising and generally having a good time – but it also massively increases the risk of almost every other disease we have already mentioned.

But don't be fooled, it's not just the old that are suffering. It's estimated that four out of five people in the UK will experience crippling back pain at some stage in their lives. (In parts of the less developed world this figure is more like 4 in 100)

Just stop and watch the way that people walk and move around on the streets and note just how far they are from the natural posture that humans should display. How many different ways of walking can you spot? Did you know that humans are the only species of animal who have this sort of variation? All other animals move in exactly the same way as same way as the rest of their species. There's no variation, except in the very old or the injured. We're not meant to slouch, stoop or shuffle: we're meant to stand upright, strong and straight but we're so dysfunctional many of us simply can't. Even children walking to school are already showing signs structural collapse – their slouched postures clearly showing their athleticism is already being severely compromised and they are setting themselves up to become just another hunched office worker of the future.

I work with people who spend all day sitting badly in chairs, gradually increasing the effect of gravity on their spine until they no longer have even one joint that has a proper range of movement. The chairbound individual is then well on the path towards an old age in which he or she is bent over so far forwards that only pulling their head well back allows them to look straight ahead. Not a good look!

So what are we doing about this?

The NHS has developed treatments for dealing with some of these ailments and diseases as and when they present themselves. Doctors are given targets to meet, so they generally treat problems with drugs or surgery, which usually alleviate the symptoms, but they aren't encouraged to spend any time thinking about preventative medicine or to take much time to consider the cause of the disease. Their training, while broad-ranging and diverse, includes barely a sidelong glance at dietary factors, exercise and preventative medicine.

What we don't have is any sort of comprehensive system for ensuring that these problems never happen in the first place. Surely, as the saying goes, an ounce of prevention is worth a pound of cure?

"If we could give every individual the right amount of nourishment and exercise, not too little and not too much, we would have found the safest way to health"
Hippocrates

At the risk of sounding too cynical, it has to be pointed out there is much more money to be made in treating diseases with fancy, expensive drugs than there is in establishing practices which keep disease at bay. There is no doubt that a preventative approach would save taxpayers' money in the long-run; however, fat-cat pharmaceutical companies would not find any such development a profitable one.

One prong for any well-organised and thought-out program to improve health and wellbeing should be to get the nation moving again. This just isn't happening at the moment for adults or for children. Provision for school sport in the UK is weak because our political masters, in their wisdom, have previously sold off our playing fields, and even today are still undermining the legislation that protects what's left. Even given

56

generous sports fields, we simply haven't left enough time in the day for sports, physical education. or play in an ever more crowded, target-driven curriculum.

National 'couch syndrome'

We have truly become a sedentary nation. In 2008, only 39% of men and 29% of women met the government's recommendation of two-and-a-half hours of exercise a week. Less than a quarter of adults now play regular sport ('regular' defined as more than 11 occasions per month). Over 44% of men are sedentary for more than six hours a day at weekends. (The figures for women are little better.)

Even for those who do exercise during the week, the benefits they gain are often undermined by poor exercise selection and practice. Most who choose a sport to keep fit fail to recognise the one-sided nature of their chosen activity and the inherent disadvantages it poses. To make matters worse, they don't see how flogging away too hard is both unnatural and can cause serious health implications. Two contrasting examples are cycling and walking.

Cycling is often touted as great all-round exercise – but it's simply not. Cycling is great for the heart, lungs and leg muscles but is next to useless for improving posture, flexibility, agility, balance or upper body strength. Many cyclists have serious mobility issues that end up with a physio referral.

Even the benefits it does offer are quickly lost if the individual overtrains by pursuing the activity in the form of heavy cardio. A long, leisurely Sunday bike ride is great. Some quick hill sprints once or twice a week – even better. But logging hundreds of miles a week in a competitive, hunched-over frenzy where the intensity means you can no longer chat easily with your riding partner is a recipe for overtraining, exhaustion and compromised health. Pushed too hard, your body will react against all your best efforts and intentions.

Another example: **walking** is fantastic exercise, working the body through chains of natural movement that have developed over millions of years. It's great basic aerobic exercise, inherently relaxing and easy on the joints. More will be said about how fantastic walking is later in the book. On its own, it's only half a programme at best, yet many people rely on it exclusively for fitness. To become truly 'all round fit' they would need to add a number of extra components, especially some specific time to **work the body closer to its full capacity for very *short* periods of time.**

Lift some weight

It is also essential that the bodies muscles are challenged to push, pull and lift heavier things on a regular basis (though body-weight exercises can be sufficient). This ensures that strength continues to develop through the 30s, 40s and maybe even well into the 50s. Thereafter, in later years, the aim is simply to hang onto as much strength and muscle mass for as long as possible. Lean muscle mass has been shown to be an excellent indicator of future health and also reduces the risk of osteoporosis (the reduced bone density that often leads to fractures and brittle bones in old age).

The take home points of this section are that exercise needs to be a rounded affair with elements chosen judiciously to balance each other. Yes, it's important to do things you like and will stick with, but too many people have little understanding of the effect that their chosen sports or exercise has on their body – especially when taken to extremes or practised, like most of us, with a badly compressed spine and poor levels of general mobility.

As depressing as it sounds, the overall analysis of the situation is that most of us simply aren't doing enough and, of those of us who are, most do not have a balanced programme that promotes long-term development, injury avoidance and overall health.

> *"If it weren't for the fact that the TV set and the refrigerator are so far apart, some of us wouldn't get any exercise at all."*
> **Joey Adam (US comedian 1911-1999)**

The glum statistics this chapter kicked off with are caused, in my opinion, by a number of key factors:

1. *Successive governments' well-meaning attempts to control our macronutrient balance (our dietary balance of calories from fat, carbs or protein) under pressure from lobby groups and industry.*

2. *A food industry quick to capitalise on producing foods we crave – but which are often doing us untold harm.*

3. *A medical industry more interested in dispensing drugs with the guidance (and financial support) of the pharmaceutical industry than actually finding and treating the underlying causes of illness.*

4. *A pharmaceutical industry focused on its own profit from selling drugs to the medical industry.*

5. *A general lifestyle that is almost devoid of the sort of movement we need to remain properly functioning human beings.*

So as you can see, there is no other person or organisation of influence that you can really trust to have your best interests as their number one consideration. The fact is, the only person who *should* have and *does* have responsibility for your overall health and wellbeing is *you.*

Key chapter points:

- *Modern diseases are becoming more common, despite medical advances in other areas.*

- *Heart disease, obesity, diabetes, cancer, stress and depression are rampant, although these diseases were totally unknown to our ancient ancestors.*

- *Muscular and skeletal issues are also increasingly common, affecting almost all adults over 30, whether or not they are aware of it yet.*

- *Those few adults and children who play regular sport offset some of the automatic damage that curse a sedentary existence. Most sports come with serious inherent drawbacks however, and few can be relied on for a total all-round fitness Programme.*

References:

1. NHS (2011) Statistics on Obesity, Physical Activity and Diet in England [Online] Available at: http://www.ic.nhs.uk/webfiles/publications/003_Health_Lifestyles/opad11/Statistics_on_Obesity_Physical_Activity_and_Diet_ England_2011_revised_Aug11.pdf

CHAPTER FOUR

A Fork in the Road

"Every human being has a two million year old man within himself; if he loses contact with that two million year old self, he loses his real roots"
Laurens Van de Post

This aim of this chapter is to give you some historical perspective: to help you understand how once healthy humans became sickly, smaller and less intelligent. Once you see where we came from and where are now, I hope you'll have a clearer idea about how we can move forward.

Let's go right, right back: back to the time when human-like species first walked out of the African forest on two legs. No-one knows for sure exactly when and why we gave up the trees for good and stopped using four limbs like a chimp. Most likely it was because of natural climate change and the disappearance of the forest and its replacement with wide-open savannah. Whatever the case it seems clear humans no longer needed to spend all their time in the trees and, after thousands of years, had evolved to the point where we were more comfortable looking for food on the ground. For the first time, humans stayed down on the savannah and began to adopt new food sources. This meant they no longer had to depend on tree-borne fruit in the way that their semi-human ancestors had.

Where once their food had been almost entirely nuts, berries, roots, fruits and vegetables that they found around them, they increasingly sourced the valuable calories and nutrients from a more concentrated source – animal meat. There was usually an abundant supply of food with natural seasonal variation. In time they learnt how to fish and, later, how to cook.

Cooking was a crucial evolutionary step, as it meant that calories could be digested more easily. Food could be eaten more quickly and less energy was used as digestion was already partly completed by the cooking process. This meant better access to the vitamins and minerals they needed, loads of calories, and lots of spare time.

With all this spare time and improved nutrition, over thousands of years our ancestors grew in stature, knowledge, language skills and development. More of their time was used for play, artistic endeavour, weapon making, and socialisation.

Greater intelligence raises a human being's chances of survival and procreation so, over the course of many millennia, an evolutionary slide towards being a species with superior intelligence was the natural result.

For the next million years or so, humans continued to grow and flourish as a species. They became bigger, cleverer, more sophisticated creatures, capable of adapting to a growing number of different habitats. They studied their environment and learnt new behaviours to better cope with new challenges. As explained earlier in the book, those incapable of such changes did not survive long enough to pass on their weaker genes through their progeny.

Each tribe or group accumulated a mass of wisdom that each passed onto the next generation through tribal wisdom, example, tradition and rite. Each new generation was taught by the older one where to fish, how to hunt, where to find edible fungi, how to build shelters; all the things needed to live life off the land.

During this time, and for most of their existence, they were nomadic or semi-nomadic. If they had 'homes' they were temporary structures or natural shelters (like caves). It was essential for them to be able to remain mobile. When the game, flora or fauna in an area became too poor, they needed to be able to move on. They may also have followed the path of migrating animals (antelope for example) and changed area according to the season. There was no obvious reason to stay in one place for very long so the whole prehistoric world was theirs to roam and explore.

A grave mistake?

All of a sudden, this undoubtedly healthy but somewhat unpredictable hunting and gathering came to a crashing halt. The discovery of a process that *appeared* to make grains digestible and the subsequent advent of large-scale farming totally upset the apple cart. For the very first time the newly discovered milling process gave humans an apparently guaranteed source of calories and the ability to *store* food in large quantities. With the possibility of starvation considerably lowered and food produced in ever-greater quantities, it was now possible to support a growing population and larger families.

In the hope of an easier life, the males gave up their hunter status to become cultivators of the land, working much longer hours and spending much of their time physically grinding grain with basic pestle and mortar equipment. Women also gave up their relaxed role as foragers in favour of rearing more children and supporting their partners on farms or smallholdings. Previously, hunted and foraged food was pretty much 'instant' and edible 'straight off the jungle floor'. With the advent of agriculture, time that was previously spent relaxing, dancing or socializing was now taken up with the extensive preparation and cooking of these new 'wonder' grains.

Farming and processing meant that previously inedible foods could now be consumed with no obvious side effects. Crops such as barley, wheat and rye simply could not have been eaten before because, as wild cereals, they have their own toxin defences that prevent them from being successfully ingested. Even animals are forced to leave them alone and search for more edible alternatives. The new milling process meant that, with lots of work, these plants could now be digested by human beings as well as fed to their cattle. This changed everything.

How do we know all this?

The science of Paleopathology studies signs of disease in ancient people. Scientists in this field are able to identify the moment the switch to agriculture took place in various parts of the world with surprising accuracy.[1] They do this by examining Paleolithic rubbish dumps where ancient excrement reveals the switch from wild plants and animals to cultivated crops. They also spend a great deal of time examining skeletons for various markers of ill health.

Skeletons reveal much more than the owner's sex, weight, and approximate age. In cases where many skeletons are found together, the expected life span and risk of death at any given age can be calculated. Paleopathologists can work out growth rates by measuring the bones of people of different ages, examining teeth for enamel defects (signs of childhood malnutrition), and recognising scars left on bones by anaemia, tuberculosis, leprosy, and other diseases.

Humans swapped their entirely edible, totally natural, foraged food sources which they had adapted to eating over millions of years to a new grain-based diet which, although more dependable, was only partially digestible. Toxins that had previously prevented grain consumption were still present, just in smaller quantities that posed less immediate danger. As well as containing toxins, these new foods also lacked much of the vital nutritional value of the forest foods they replaced.

It is clear that adopting grains as a mainstay had a truly devastating effect on our species. Within a comparatively small amount of time the records show that humans developed a brand new range of miserable diseases they had never before faced; they also grew shorter in stature and, with an exploding population, became utterly dependent on farmed land for their survival.

Professor Jared Diamond of the University of California, winner of the US National Medal of Science, points out that one measurable factor that tells us a lot about the health of a given race of people is height:

Skeletons from Greece and Turkey show that the average height of hunger-gatherers toward the end of the ice ages was a generous 5' 9" for men, 5' 5" for women. With the adoption of agriculture, height crashed, and by 3000 B. C. had reached a low of only 5' 3" for men, 5' for women. By classical times heights were very slowly on the rise again, but modern Greeks and Turks have still not regained the average height of their distant ancestors.

Another example of paleopathology at work is the study of Indian skeletons from burial mounds in the Illinois and Ohio river valleys. At Dickson Mounds, located near the confluence of the Spoon and Illinois rivers, archaeologists have excavated some 800 skeletons that paint a picture of the health changes that occurred when a hunter-gatherer culture gave way to intensive maize farming around A. D. 1150. Studies by George Armelagos and his colleagues then at the University of Massachusetts show these early farmers paid a price for their new-found livelihood. Compared to the hunter-gatherers who preceded them, the farmers had a nearly 50 per cent increase in enamel defects indicative of malnutrition, a fourfold increase in iron-deficiency anemia (evidenced by a bone condition called porotic hyperostosis), a threefold rise in bone lesions reflecting infectious disease in general, and an increase in degenerative conditions of the spine, probably reflecting a lot of hard physical labor. "Life expectancy at birth in the pre-agricultural community was about twenty-six years," says Armelagos, "but in the post-agricultural community it was nineteen years. So these episodes of nutritional stress and infectious disease were seriously affecting their ability to survive."

~ Professor Jared Diamond, "The Worst Mistake in the History of the Human Race," Discover Magazine, May 1987, pp. 64-66

The trade-off for this new way of life was considerable. So great, in fact, that some thinkers consider the advent of agriculture to be the greatest mistake our race has ever made. Professor Diamond makes a brilliant case for this in his book, *Guns, Germs and Steel*.[2]

The main reason for these perhaps shocking findings is that while hunter-gatherers enjoyed a varied diet, early farmers obtained most of their food from just a few starchy crops. These early agriculturalists gained cheap, reliable calories but at the cost of poor nutrition. They concentrated their efforts on producing high-yield, high-carbohydrate crops like rice and potatoes, whereas the mix of wild plants and animals in the diets of surviving hunter-gatherers provided more protein, vitamins, minerals and essential fatty acids. The nomads therefore enjoyed a better balance of essential nutrients – not to mention a more relaxed lifestyle.

(Today, by the way, just three high-carbohydrate plants – wheat, rice, and corn – provide the bulk of the calories consumed by the human species, yet each one is deficient in vitamins and amino acids essential to life. Certainly, in the 21st century, we eat a more varied diet than these early farmers, but these high-carbohydrate plants still represent the vast majority of our calories.)

Despite the initial lure of an easier life, these farmers were in fact forced to work much harder than hunter-gatherers to survive. They would perform manual labour (which you might think would keep them fit) but without sufficient recovery time it meant that, like the marathon runners we mentioned earlier, the toll on their health was great.

For comparison, we have a good idea of how hard our hunter-gatherer ancestors worked because scattered across the world there are several dozen groups of so-called primitive people, like the Kalahari Bushmen or the Hadza of Tanzania, who continue to support themselves in a way that has remained unchanged throughout history. These people have plenty of leisure time, sleep a good deal, and work less hard than their farming neighbours. For instance, the average time devoted to obtaining food is only 12 to 19 hours a week for the Bushmen, while the nomadic Hadza work for fewer than 14 hours.

Early farmers, by contrast, worked most or all of the daylight hours and possibly after dark too, by candlelight.

You might expect that eventually humans would evolve to cope with this new way of living, and this new, partially toxic food matter. However, for evolution to change anything it has to change the propensity for an animal to die before it can pass on its genes to its offspring. Farming didn't do this.

In fact, farming ensured that many of the natural dangers that befell semi-nomadic man were removed from the range of possible early deaths. They were also less likely to die early as a result of starvation. Less genetically gifted human beings were now able to survive and pass their genes onto a new generation. This was effectively the end of large-scale evolutionary improvement for the human race as selection pressure was completely removed from the population. (The idea that our DNA today is identical to that of our primal ancestors is supported by hundreds of leading anthropologists, evolutionary biologists and genetic researchers[3]).

Instead, farming meant that most adults were able to stay alive long enough to procreate and then, maybe 10 years later, in their 30s, would die of one of the many diseases that attacked their weakened immune systems and prematurely-aged bodies. In this way, no evolutionary preference for 'good digesters of grains' could ever be established.

Many more people were now surviving, but they were doing no more than struggling through a growing list of ailments to what we would call early middle age. They would have been lucky to see their children reach the end of their teens.

It's important to remember that, in evolutionary terms, this trend towards grain cultivation is a flash in the pan. If the history of the human race, to put it on a simple scale, began at midnight, and we've just finished our first day on the earth, then only in last four seconds have we stopped being hunter-gatherers in favour of mass-produced agriculture. However obvious a fuel source grain might seem to us in the 21st century, it has only been a consumable option for a tiny fraction of our time on this planet.

The evidence seems to suggest that we are paying a very dear price for these last few seconds.

Another key, but arguably less dramatic moment was the arrival of the **Industrial Revolution**. Many people were freed from the need to work on small farms in the production of food. Instead, the century of the factory was upon us. Men, women and children looked to factories to survive. Ignoring the titled aristocracy and those who served them, there were two types of people: those who owned factories and those who worked in them. The huge majority fell into the second camp.

Conditions in factories were so grim (as they still are in much of the third world) that a life toiling in the fields in the sunlight in contact with nature could only be regarded as a rustic idyll. Painters and poets of the Romantic period depicted idealised scenes of country folk living simple but worthy lives, while their city-bound cousins were as cooped up and maltreated as a modern battery hen. Cramped conditions and overcrowding led to stress, disease and further malnutrition.

Only with the most recent of our revolutions have we been saved from the miserable fate that befell the common man. The **Technological Revolution** meant that factories became automated and a majority of people were paid for their ability to provide a service, communicate, create or teach. All of this can be done without the concentrated manual labour that had been a feature of working lives in the past.

At the same time, our domestic lives have also changed forever. We no longer need to wash our clothes by hand or walk to the shops; no firewood needs collecting; the lawn can be mown by an electric machine and the tree in the garden can be taken down with a chainsaw.

With new technology we no longer needed to use our bodies for most common household tasks. In fact we now need put in no more physical labour at home than we do in the work place.

Meanwhile, the complexity of our lives has increased. More technology means more opportunities, which mean more learning, which means more pressure – for both adults and children. Increasingly, schooling has had to become more intensive to ensure basic mastery of the complex skills we need to find a position in the workforce. This means that there is less time and fewer daylight hours available for children to run, jump and play as they have done for millennia. Added to this, a preference for entertainment based around technology (such as television, games consoles and mobile phones) means that even if they have the time, many children no longer have the inclination for physical play that they once did.

The Technological Revolution meant that, on top of a high-calorie, high-carb diet, many of the modern generation live a lifestyle devoid of any physical endeavour at all. It also meant that new, heavily processed foods entered our diet in concentrations that our bodies have not evolved to cope with.

Here in the 21st century, all this has caught up with us. Clearly we can't just turn back the clock in some sort of revisionist, Luddite manner (though this might still happen if we run out of oil, as my dad likes to point out!) but there must be a better alternative to the path of madness we now tread.

Here is the problem as I see it:

We are human beings living in a radically different, modern world – but our unchanged Stone Age genes expect the same challenges and environment that our ancient ancestors faced.

Our lives have changed, but our bodies and our natural instincts haven't evolved to keep up. We are Stone Age people living in the age of the microchip – no wonder we feel overwhelmingly out of place. This mismatch between gene and environment expresses itself in discomfort, disease, and compromised health and happiness.

What Darwin taught us

The theory of evolution posits the idea that natural selection will favour those people (or, more accurately, genes; c.f. *The Selfish Gene*, Richard Dawkins, 1976) who possess traits that allow them to survive and breed where others will fail. In this way, human beings have adapted over millennia to their environment – psychologically, physiologically and genetically speaking – and have made a comfortable match.

Our ancestors evolved over millions of years under very specific environmental conditions. The foods they ate, the amount of sun they got, and the sort of movement that was required of them to survive shaped their very genome. Over the past 10,000 years, the world has changed in innumerable ways, for both better and worse, but the human genome has changed very little. Simply put, if mankind wants a happy, healthy future – might we be better off looking back to our past?

Over the last few thousand years, lifestyles have changed far more rapidly than evolution has been able to keep up with.

It is clear that humans are no longer perfectly adapted to their environment: backs hurt from sitting in chairs; eyes weaken from close reading all day; legs and arms waste from little exercise and stomachs grow from an abundance of cheap, empty calories.

We have changed our environment so quickly that although our high-tech lives appear much easier, there is a hidden price to pay in each deviation from the lifestyle we are genetically predisposed to expect.

This isn't an idealistic endorsement for grabbing a club or spear and re-enacting a cave-dweller's lifestyle, so much as considering the conditions and demands a cave dweller's body would have known, and using them as a template from which to produce an optimal template for health. This essentially means *doing* the very things that *promoted* their wellness, fat burning, muscle building and longevity and *avoiding* the things that still cause fat storing, muscle wastage, disease and illness.

Key chapter points:

- *Evidence suggests that humans became shorter, weaker and less healthy when they abandoned the life of the hunter-gatherer to cultivate crops.*

- *The Industrial Revolution meant we could produce new crops on a huge scale. People had to work in the factories or fields for long hours.*

- *The Technological Revolution means that humans now have little reason to exert themselves or even move about much. A sedentary existence has ushered in a host of new problems.*

- *Little movement, when combined with a processed high-carb diet has partially crippled much of the western world. Our genes expect movement, real food and an outdoor life.*

- *The government's attempts to help have often been hopelessly misplaced.*

References

1. Mummert A et al. (2011) "Stature and robusticity during the agricultural transition: evidence from the bioarchaeological record." Economics and Human Biology 9:284-301.

2. Diamond J (2005) Guns, *Germs, and Steel: The Fates of Human Societies*, WW Norton, New York.

3. For example, see the work of Dr. Boyd Eaton, chief anthropologist at Emory University in Atlanta and author of *The Paleo Prescription* and James V. Neel, of the University of Michigan's Department of Genetics.

CHAPTER FIVE

"Instinctive Fitness" – A Third Way

"The wise man sees in the misfortune of others what he himself should avoid"
Marcus Aurelius
(Roman Emperor 121-180)

Of course it's probably not exactly breaking news to you to hear that sitting around all day and doing little exercise is bad for our health. Moving is what our bodies yearn to do and by keeping them still all the time they are cheated of the stimulus they need to function properly.

You might rightfully ask how Instinctive Fitness is different to anything you've heard before, and why this approach differs to what you may have tried in the past. To answer this we're going to look closer at the uncomfortable introduction that most of us have to the world of physical exercise, examine the unhelpful assumptions that modern exercise is based upon, and look at the background and history that makes today's 'keep fit' culture the painful experience it often is.

A sorry introduction to movement and exercise

Movement and exercise are two of the biggest factors in daily life about which we've all been completely led astray by so-called 'experts'. We've been convinced that fitness and strength come only through prolonged pain and hardship – to the point that the mere utterance of the word 'exercise' or 'get fit' sends a shudder through many a heart.

Far too many people instantly conjure up painful and sometimes traumatic childhood memories of their last failed foray into the world of 'shorts, T-shirts and gym shoes'. Typically our first (and sometimes only) brush with structured, physical exercise begins aged 5 in school 'gym' or 'games' classes.

71

Now if you were one of the competitive kids who really liked organised sport or formal gym, then physical education lessons were probably a useful introduction to a lifetime of health and activity. It was more than likely the highlight of your week; a session you found fun and looked forward to. Everybody enjoys activities that come naturally to them and they will keep coming back for more. But unfortunately, for many other children, it was certainly a very different story.

Many kids just *hate* the style of physical education served up in school: they loathe being lumped together and dread having to run round with other fitter, more physical pupils. They detest having their apparent physical inadequacies and lack of coordination paraded before the world. Many wrongly decide at a very early age that they are obviously physically inferior and that exercise is not for them. An emotional, spur of the moment decision – perhaps triggered by one single, fleetingly bad experience – can result in them jumping to a wrong conclusion at an age when they really shouldn't be making such life-changing decisions.

As an adult, if you find something that's not right for you, you have the option to leave it; to walk away and perhaps come back at a later date. For school children it was (and still is) a totally different scenario. They have no option but to run the painful gauntlet of the physical education lesson, regardless of their fear, humiliation and discomfort.

The problem is aggravated because 'games' teachers probably loved their subject when they were children, and simply don't understand those children who don't feel the same way. Like any other more academic subject, teachers are understandably confused and frustrated by those students who don't throw themselves into their pet subject with the same enthusiasm. The feeling of marginalisation that these children experience in class can last a lifetime and exerts heavy toll on attitudes towards sport, fitness and all physical activity in general.

It is such a shame that bad experiences at school lead to a large percentage of the adult population closing the door on the joy of physical movement and exercise at a very early age. At the very moment they are able to leave school, many stop exercising – and plenty never return.

Exercise *must* hurt – mustn't it?

Let's face it; once our instinctive and very natural taste for running, jumping, lifting and stretching has been cast aside, there are few incentives offered by the health and fitness industries to entice anyone back.

Other than the negative guilt served up by the government, press and media, there outwardly appears to be little pleasurable about exercise. How could there be when every workout video, every training DVD, every drill-sergeant-style boot camp screams *'No pain, no gain!'* and *'Feel the burn!'?*

Who in their right mind would ever choose to put their hand up and eagerly *shout: "Oh me, me! I'll have some of that exquisite torture please"*?

The reality is that exercise should never hurt

Except under very brief and controlled conditions that we'll cover later, nature intended exercise (i.e. natural human movement) to be stimulating, enjoyable and invigorating – never painful. Of course, if you want to become a competitive international athlete, this clear-cut picture does blur somewhat, but for the man or woman in the street who wants...

- *Greater strength*

- *More energy*

- *Better stamina*

- *More flexibility*

- *Better balance*

- *Greater speed*

- *And more power*

*...getting fit does not **ever** need to make you sweat profusely, puff, pant, wheeze or endure 'stitches' and joint and muscle pain.*

The problem with the traditional, hard-line school of thought is that it puts most people off from coming back and trying exercise ever again. It's quite obviously not intentional – why would an industry want to deliberately alienate its customers? It's just that it's what the exercise 'experts' themselves have been taught. It's all they know. It's not only written into their professional curriculum, it's written into everybody's shared history and consciousness.

A tiny bit of 'modern' history

Societies going back as far as the ancient Greeks, the Spartans and the Romans recognised the importance of adding a regime of exercise to the daily grind. Physical training was held in high esteem by a whole host of cultures that developed various methods of offsetting the damage caused by lifestyles that were becoming increasingly sedentary and comfortable. What they all had in common was a requirement for battle-ready soldiers and a strong civilian population ready to fight to preserve their freedom if called upon. If soft civilians were the problem, tough training was the answer.

No matter what their area of expertise, today 99% of physical training 'experts' can trace their fundamental principles and their professional history back to this sort of very regimented and specialised *military* training.

Today, military-style "boot camps" are enjoying a strange new lease of life, as sedentary people sign-up to have their independence handed over to a shouting instructor who will repeatedly and repetitively cajole, push and harry them through the pain barrier and past their reluctance to engage in any movement at all. They are encouraged to put their freedom, their feelings of comfort, and their natural sense for what's good for them to one side, and surrender to the painful routine their well-meaning instructor has lined up.

The drill sergeant in disguise

It's clear why training has developed like this. This form of exercise was (and still is) part and parcel of the breaking down of civilians and the building up of 'battle-ready' soldiers. Tyrannical drill sergeants are tasked with 'beasting' soft, lazy and undisciplined 'raw' recruits into supremely fit and regimented warriors in a matter of weeks. This means that for the military, exercise is not only the road to physical fitness, but a big stick with which to beat the tardy civilian into a new, fearsome 'fighting machine' able to unhesitatingly obey orders and overcome any level of discomfort.

Back when Britain had colonial wars to win, a gradual, gentle, natural road to fitness was never going to deliver the required result in good time, and few of these wars were ever going to be won by an army that made virtue of 'taking it easy' and respecting their bodies' limits.

A new, tougher approach was needed that would push both the recruits' bodies and minds further than nature ever intended. Stress, injury and health be damned – what was required here was an intensity

74

of training that, to all intents and purposes, shattered the independent spirit who unwittingly took the King's shilling. This dehumanising process was necessary to build up the red breasted, man-shaped 'war machine' the armed forces required. Given its purpose, this pretty brutal style of physical and mental training was enormously successful, producing the sort of military might that helped forge an empire 'upon which the sun never set'. For better or worse, by 1922 a quarter of the globe was shaded pink and under British rule.

Unfortunately, although this sort of fitness regime is great for moulding soldiers quickly, it's a complete disaster as a long-term personal fitness strategy. You certainly *can* get soldiers fit in a few weeks with these methods, especially if you're not worried about breaking a few on the way. However, keeping this intensity up for longer than a few months is actually impossible and will always result in exhaustion, injury and ill-health over the longer term. Even the military doesn't try. After six weeks or so of exhausting strife, and after the culmination of their basic training, their fitness is maintained mostly by actually doing the job in hand, now a base level of fitness and unity of team spirit has been established.

Any type of military-inspired training camp is a very different kettle of fish indeed to a sustainable lifetime of self-motivated, natural and enjoyable physical activity. But that didn't stop these drill sergeants – the only 19th century health and fitness experts – from exporting their extensive 'know how' away from the drill square to the outside world.

Army boots and webbing turn into gym vests and plimsolls

Long before there was an established, accredited 'health and leisure' industry, many British public schools (as the oldest private schools in the UK are known) with regimental ties took a role in preparing their young charges for a more-than-likely career in military service. Later, when grammar and comprehensive schools were established, many adopted the 'games' and training techniques of these older schools into their own curriculum. In time, both the ethos and methods of military training permeated through society to reach everybody and become the only accepted route to physical fitness. A training style that was possible only for a few weeks at a time – and only really suitable for moulding soldiers into fighting units – became the accepted approach for everyone, even those looking for a sustainable, effective, enjoyable approach to exercise that would last a lifetime. In this way, military-style physical training slipped into our schools and then into all of our lives by the back door.

And so the die was cast: Fitness and health wrongly became synonymous with pain, with graft, with labour and with toil.

Underneath the lycra

Sure, if this shouting, screaming, gnashing of teeth road to fitness floats your boat, then by all means sign on the dotted line and pay someone to thrash you into shape. There's loads of choice: underneath the enticing and attractive lycra, leg warmers, Nike shoes and smile of your modern 'spinning', Boxercise and Zumba classes – still beats the steely heart of 19th century military tyrant.

If however, physical pain is not your cup of tea, then it might be time for you to look for another gentler, yet more effective alternative – and fortunately, you've come to just the right place.

From one extreme to the other

Before we move on, let's take a quick look at various people's current relationship with physical exercise…

It's pretty much a given that everyone 'knows' they should be fit and healthy, and nearly everyone, if given the choice, would *choose* to be fit and healthy. Some people put the care and maintenance of their body at the centre of their lifestyle, open-mindedly exploring what works best for them. Others blindly go through the motions they've been told are right and not noticing they're getting nowhere fast.

Others just don't seem to give a…

For much of the population, health and fitness seems to be a chore to be ignored, avoided or a luxury continually pushed to one side. The following categories are of course generalisations, and few people fit neatly into just one camp, but I think people can, by and large, be fairly neatly divided into just two groups.

1. The sedentary time bomb (doesn't care – or tries not to)

The first option is filled with apathetic individuals who are generally doing nothing other than what life actively demands. This means that, for the most part, they are taking it easy, moving very little at all and indulging heavily in 'bait foods', which fool us with their attractive but manufactured appearance and taste.

These people take the common position of assuming that if everyone else does little exercise and eats foods full of sugar and starch, then it's okay for them to do so too (as long as the saturated fats are kept under control of course!)

This may be OK for the first few decades, but as the years and pounds roll on – heart disease, diabetes, cancer and all the other health monsters wait patiently in the wings before arriving on stage to play major roles in the rest of their life.

2. The fitness martyr ('No pain, no gain')

The second option is for people who not only want to be in better shape – but also are actually prepared to do something about it. This is a path the vast majority seem to take. On and off at least.

Usually set off by listening to a friend, reading a magazine or buying a book or DVD that spurs them into action, this person has all the best intentions to shape up. So they roll up their sleeves and prepare themselves for the hard slog they're going to put themselves through. This new found enthusiasm usually lasts a few weeks or even months, usually with one sole intention in mind – to fit into a new dress, look 'buff' on the beach holiday or look good in upcoming wedding photos.

This intense campaign is normally based around a new diet with an emphasis on consuming fewer calories (assuming that weight loss is a goal), perhaps accompanied by an exercise routine of some sort, frequently featuring the 'regular' use of a gym with its array of resistance and cardio machines.

Sometimes, through following a regime like this the stated goals can indeed be met (e.g. lose 9 pounds of fat by March); more often, however, they're not. More likely, the trainee strays from the path they've set themselves and fails to see the programme through to the end.

Whether or not these goals are met, the usual pattern is that after a certain amount of time our once-keen dieter and exerciser returns to their previous habits. Sooner rather than later, the individual finds themselves back in the condition they were in before they started their programme: Any pounds that were lost are quickly regained and, more often than not, a few more pounds are added to take the belt out one more hole. Any benefits of all the hardship are quickly buried beneath a new malaise of inactivity. The individual then feels the shame of having failed to reach their goals.

We've all been there right?

They will get over their failure in time and – sooner or later – will begin another project of self-improvement based on the deluded hope that they can summon higher levels of will power this time round, or that a little tweaking to their programme will make all the difference.

Remember what Einstein said about continuing to do the same thing but expecting different results? I'd like to suggest that there is a third way; a third option that avoids the folly of the two most common approaches to fitness and health.

Instinctive Fitness – the third way

OK, I'm going to hold my hands up here and admit this won't all happen without some changes to your lifestyle. There is no magical silver bullet that will banish the pounds, build the muscle and present you with greater health for nothing. But this is also not just another fad regime – temporary and probably useless. Instead, 'instinctive' fitness offers a philosophy to help you adopt *the* most natural way of getting into and maintaining a great level of fitness.

Of course some effort will be needed to get started. You're probably going to have to roll your sleeves up for the first 30 days, stick to the rules like glue. After that you can let the fact that exercise is now more fun and food is actually tastier, along with the pleasure you take in looking and feeling fantastic, carry you along with its own momentum.

The biggest incentive though is that, should you choose to take on the challenge for just 30 days, you will never want to stray back to your old habits. It actually gets easier as the weeks roll by, not harder. You really won't be counting the days until you can get back to 'normal', as eating and exercising 'instinctively' becomes a very welcome, very natural part of your life.

A natural fitness

By banishing all the hardships, stresses and strains intrinsic to any other 'fad' diets, eating plenty of genuinely satisfying food and by exercising in ways, easier and more fun than you've probably ever known – fitness and health really can be maintained effortlessly. Once the first 30 days are out of the way, 'instinctive' fitness is actually an easier habit to maintain than returning to the alternative 'time bomb' or the martyr's way of living.

Getting in shape – and *staying* in shape – shouldn't involve Herculean amounts of effort or the will power of Ghandi. The approach to take is one of sustainable, long-term change. The basic rule is:

Make Small, Comfortable Changes You Can Keep Up Forever.

Therefore, what I'm proposing is neither a diet (which has a ring of the temporary about it right from the outset) nor a programme of frantic activity with a beginning and an end. Instead, Instinctive Fitness is an immensely enjoyable and rewarding **Lifestyle**.

'Instinctive' fitness is about making minor lifestyle changes that are so painless, so easy to follow, so rewarding and offer such life enhancing results that it's easy to keep them up forever.

That isn't to say that either you or I won't ever overindulge ourselves again, as we surely will; but the difference when keeping yourself fit 'instinctively' is that you'll feel great when you do and worse when you don't; and if you do succumb to temptation you'll actually look forward to getting back on track straight away.

Nobody is suggesting that the transition will be really, really easy. However, once the switch has been made, there's little effort needed to keep going, and little incentive to turn back the clock to old habits. You will have developed a new instinct that should see you good for the rest of your life.

Role models

I believe it can be helpful to develop some new models of fitness to inspire us and realign us with our best intentions.

To do this, I'm not going to suggest any famous Austrian Bodybuilders (either in their prime or their embarrassing flabby, coronary-challenged present), or media personalities such as Brad Pitt or Jenifer Aniston whom people admire for their beautifully presented (airbrushed) bodies. This is simply because:

Instinctive Fitness shouldn't be all about what you look like.

I'd like to offer you some alternative role models who offer a beauty and depth greater than your average catwalk model or boy band member. These are people with not only an admirable level of physical capacity but also a strength of character that makes them the embodiment of our most primitive and glorious human spirit.

1. Gymnasts and decathletes/heptathletes

The UK, in 2012 was a great year for the British Olympic team and whose medalists included people who really can be considered among the kings and queens of modern athletes.

Pro: an incredible bodyweight-to-strength ratio, speed, endurance, flexibility, co-ordination, balance, focus and concentration, great agility and low body-fat; also, there's very little 'chronic cardio' in their programme. Jessica Ennis should be an inspiration for anyone.

Con: They work out for many exhausting hours a day; the female gymnasts often have poor posture from having to pose with a backward leaning spine on completing difficult landings; too many females eat poorly (and like mice) in order to keep their statures small and light-weight.

2. Warriors

Choose whatever image of warrior is most powerful for you. Think of the greatest warriors from any time or place whose fitness was a product of their lifestyle. For women, the image of the warrior queen or that of the Amazonian women can be a helpful one.

Pro: Strength, endurance, speed, spontaneity of movement, power, awareness, balance, patience, ability to adapt.

Con: Not all warriors are as mobile, flexible and injury resistant as they should be. A lesser breed depends too heavily on sheer strength rather than quality and speed of movement. Regimented soldiers suffer from repetitive stress injuries and overtraining far too often.

3. The caveman or cavewoman (my favourite, of course!)

A thoroughbred human with no catch net in life: Someone who lives (and dies) on their physicality and wits in a way the modern 'civilised' world can no longer understand. Like the warrior, their fitness emerges naturally from their lifestyle.

Pro: Resilient, strong, stamina-filled, 100% natural human movement patterns, health, explosive speed, awareness of environment, low-body fat, high body-to-weight ratio.

Con: Might have been short of nutrients during very hard times; had to endure the cold and some hardship; depended on their hunting skills, wits and instincts to survive.

If it helps to hold one of these models in your mind, or perhaps any other type of character who can truly inspire you, then please do so – perhaps even 'Google' a few images to place on your desktop?

Alternatively, you might choose a modern individual to inspire you. You might choose **Bruce Lee**, who had one leg-shorter than the other, was badly short-sighted, bullied as a child, shorter than average height, of mixed race, and had damaged his back so badly he was told he'd never kick again. However, none of this stopped him becoming the greatest martial artist ever and the first ever Asian Hollywood star.

Or you might choose someone more down-to-earth such as **Jack LaLanne,** the US fitness guru who, aged 70, handcuffed, shackled, and fighting strong winds and currents, swam 1 mile towing 70 rowboats, one containing several guests, from the Queen's Way Bridge in the Long Beach Harbour to the Queen Mary.[1]

You could look into the lifestyle of **Professor Art de Vany**, who (on a Paleo diet) trains by pushing and pulling his Range Rover up and down his drive. Art is 70 years old and has less than 8% body fat (which is about the same as a professional bodybuilder).

Or, more recently and closer to home, consider the achievements of **Eddie Izzard** who ran around the perimeter of the UK in seven weeks in 2009 with back-to-back marathons; or **David Walliams** who swam the length of the Thames in 2010. Both of these comedians (what is it about comedians?) were fairly sedentary until they put their minds to their new challenges. Of course I can't really recommend Izzard's extreme endurance feats, but I can't help admiring his courage and total dedication to the task.

These specific models of health and vitality may – or may not – be a perfect inspiration to you, but are presented to help you recognise real physical potency when compared to the false aesthetic of the skinny (but unhealthy and weak) catwalk model.

Here are a few questions for you to consider. For most of these questions, if the answer is a no, then an imperative should have been set-up – turn this to a yes.

Real world fitness test

1. *Could you jump a five foot ditch (perhaps even from standing)?*

2. *Could you climb a tree to rescue an animal or stuck child, or perhaps evade an animal?*

3. *Could you hurdle a garden gate if the hinge was stuck?*

4. *Could you carry an adult out of a burning building?*

5. *Could you get to the top floor of a sixth-storey building, taking the steps at a run, two at a time?*

6. *Could you run for a bus at 90% of the top speed you have ever reached in your whole life?*

7. *Could you drag a heavy fallen branch off the road?*

If you find yourself saying: "Yeah, right – at my age!" then you've bought into the prevailing myth of degeneration with time. I know individuals in their 70s who can (or could if required) do all of these things.

These questions are all about real world abilities that make our lives greater for their presence, and those abilities that, in times of peril, will change people's lives forever. This is what real fitness should be about, and is clearly a very different prospect than the mere LOOK of fitness.

Perhaps bearing these kinds of endeavour in mind will keep the coming challenges real. Maybe you'll never quite manage all of these achievements; however, there's accomplishment in every inch you move in this direction, and there's the satisfaction of knowing your ambitions are for real world ends.

All-round health

Any personal measurement of health is of course subjective – so if you think you *feel* fit and healthy then you must be doing at least something right. But *real* fitness really should go beyond subjective personal opinions such as:

- *Immunity ('Oh I haven't been ill for years y'know')*

- *Energy ('I just feel so much perkier these days')*

- *Anti-ageing ('Bet you thought I was in my 30s?')*

- *Absence of pain ('Nothing hurts!')*

- *Mental health ('I'm coming down off the bridge now!')*

These are, of course, each a fine 'result' – but they are also impossible to quantify.

Instead seek very clear markers of health that professionals now consistently rely on for a more scientific picture of the body's true resilience.

These markers include:

- *resting heart-rate*

- *blood-glucose levels*

- *blood pressure*

- *body fat percentage (or hip-to-waist ratio)*

- *bone density*

- *hormonal balance*

- *lipid levels.*

*Only by working clo*ser with doctors are we ever going to persuade the general public and the wider medical community that there really is a better option when it comes to healthy living. With specific data, we can together demonstrate the universal application of a more instinctive approach to eating and exercise.

So get yourself along to your GP and get a check-up to make sure you're ready to face the coming challenge – which will also give you a baseline against which to measure future progress.

The proof of the pudding...

So far there is massive anecdotal evidence for the efficacy of the ideas being put forward; there is also a logical, anthropological reasoning, and well-documented (but ultimately scattered) research to back it all up. What there isn't enough of at the moment is consensus of opinion and mainstream recognition.

By contacting your doctor and getting as many relevant tests done as possible, you will reinforce your awareness of your own success and demonstrate the soundness of these principles to the wider community.

> *"I have the body of an eighteen year old.*
> *I keep it in the fridge".*
> **Spike Milligan**

Key chapter points:

- *There's a third way that stands apart from harmful sedentary habits and the profitless way many people spend their time trying to reach their fitness goals.*

- *It works with our own nature, our Stone Age bodies, and our unaltered genetic blueprint to bypass our too-often fragile willpower.*

- *Good models for fitness are gymnasts, warriors and pre-historic humans.*

- *Real world tests and challenges are better than counting repetitions.*

- *You only need to do 3 things well: "Move Well, Eat Well, Live Well".*

References:

1. *Wikipedia (2012) Jack LaLanne [Online] Available at:* http://en.wikipedia.org/wiki/Jack_LaLanne

CHAPTER SIX

Natural Movement

"Motion is Life"
Hippocrates

Running, jumping, climbing, skipping? So what? Why should any of us move about too much when we simply don't need to anymore? Aren't cars, buses, trains, escalators, TV remote controls and even stair lifts increasingly happy to take the strain?

So let's start right from the beginning with a dumb question: "Why do we need to move at all?"

The answer is so simple, so straightforward and so fundamental we are each in danger of overlooking it in search of something more convoluted or 'highbrow'.

*"...because movement **is** life."*

If we are unsure of something's status as a living thing, the first thing we look for is movement. The more self-directed movement we see in a creature (or plant), the more we can be sure it is indeed alive. Movement, whether we are talking about the contraction of capillaries squeezing blood around our bodies or the twitching of a suspiciously still caterpillar's leg, is the stuff of life. To a very real extent, the amount of life left in a thing can be measured by its capacity to move.

As humans, once we start to 'slow down' or to 'take life easy' (all euphemisms for sitting on one's arse more), we begin an inevitable slow degradation in physical ability, and ultimately the foreshortening of life begins.

"So many older people, they just sit around all day long and they don't get any exercise. Their muscles atrophy, and they lose their strength, their energy and vitality by inactivity".
Jack LaLanne

85

Humans engage in many different types of movement. Some of these movements are **involuntary** (such as the beating of your heart, or the inhalation of air); some are **voluntary** (skipping down the road with joy, maybe); some are of **necessity** (climbing the stairs or carrying groceries); some are for **pleasure** (dancing on a Saturday night); and some are a matter of pure **self-discipline** (most workout programmes). Perhaps a final category is **resistance of movement** (this includes, but is not limited to, the largely subconscious fight against gravity that good balance and posture involves).

If movement is life, then looking to improve the quantity and quality of all of our movement has to be the cornerstone of any approach to a better and longer time spent on Earth.

Earlier in the book we looked at the idea that much of what plagues modern humans comes out of a mismatch between their modern environment (and modern sedentary habits) and the confused instincts of the Stone Age body we all inhabit.

Perhaps not surprisingly, we don't know *exactly* what ancient hunter-gatherers did from day to day, but we do have a pretty good idea. We have a fairly clear picture for two reasons. Firstly, anthropologists have devoted hundreds of lifetimes (collectively) to studying evidence of the daily lives of ancient people, closely examining the everyday objects and rubbish they have left behind.

Secondly, our most accurate indicator of how ancient humans lived comes from anthropologists who have gone and lived with modern hunter-gatherer tribes. Their first-hand accounts of people living an unchanged existence essentially since Paleolithic times shine a bright light on what our ancestors would have got up to day-to-day.

We briefly mentioned the Hiwi and Ache people right back in Chapter Two who are still deeply embedded in nature, living in remote parts of the world even today. Dr. Kim Hill, an anthropologist at Arizona State University has spent 30 years living with and studying the Ache hunter-gatherers of Paraguay and the Hiwi foragers of South-western Venezuela. He got to know them pretty well and his description below represents a rare first-hand glimpse into the activity that would have been required of us all, were it not for modern industry and the Agricultural Revolution.

The Ache hunted every day of the year if it didn't rain...GPS data I collected...suggests that about 10 km per day is probably closer to their average distance covered during [food] searches. They might cover another 1-2 km per day in very rapid pursuit. Sometimes pursuits can be extremely strenuous and last more than an hour. Ache hunters often take an easy day after any particularly difficult day, and rainfall forces them to take a day or two a week with only an hour or two of exercise. Basically they do moderate days most of the time, and sometimes really hard days usually followed by a very easy day. The difficulty of the terrain is really what killed me (ducking under low branches and vines about once every 20 seconds all day long, and climbing over fallen trees, moving through tangled thorns etc.) I was often drenched in sweat within an hour of leaving camp, and usually didn't return for 7-9 hours with not more than 30 minutes rest during the day.

The Hiwi on the other hand only hunted about 2-3 days a week and often told me they wouldn't go out on a particular day because they were 'tired'. They would stay home and work on tools, etc. Their travel was not as strenuous as among the Ache (they often canoed to the hunt site), and their pursuits were usually shorter. But the Hiwi sometimes did amazing long distance walks that would have really hurt the Ache. They would walk to visit another village maybe 80-100 km away and then stay for only an hour or two before returning. This often included walking all night long as well as during the day. When I hunted with Machiguenga, Yora, Yanomamo Indians in the 1980s, my focal man days were much, much easier than with the Ache. And virtually all these groups take an easy day after a particularly difficult one.

While hunter gatherers are generally in good physical condition if they haven't yet been exposed to modern diseases and diets that come soon after permanent outside contact, I would not want to exaggerate their abilities. They are what you would expect if you took a genetic cross section of humans and put them in lifetime physical training at moderate to hard levels. Most hunting is search time not pursuit, thus a good deal of aerobic long distance travel is often involved (over rough terrain and carrying loads if the hunt is successful). I used to train for marathons as a grad student and could run at a 6:00 per mile pace for 10 miles, but the Ache would run me into the ground following peccary tracks through dense bush for a couple of hours.

In a separate account of the behaviours of the Paraguayan Ache population Dr. Hill reported:

On a foraging trip, camp members rise early, eat whatever is left over from the previous day, and set out in search of food. The men lead the way, carrying only bows and arrows, and women and children follow, the women carrying young children and the family's possessions in a woven basket. Some men walk with their wives and carry children on their shoulders. The foragers do not walk on trails but break a new path through the forest each day. Usually the leaders set out in the direction of an area known or thought to contain important food resources. After walking together for about an hour, the two sexes separate, with men walking further and more rapidly in search of game, and women and children slowly progressing in the general direction the men have set out. Men generally eat very little during the day, but women and children sometimes collect and eat fruits and insects while men hunt, and women often process palm trunks for their starchy fibre near the end of the day. This snacking usually' accounts for less than 5% of all food consumed (Hill et al. 1981).

All camp members come together again at the end of the day, when they clear a small camp in the underbrush, build fires, and prepare and share food extensively. Evening is considered the most pleasant time, with band members enjoying their only large meal of the day, and joking and singing in the night. While in the forest the Ache sleep on the ground or on palm-leaf mats in a small circle. They build palm-leaf huts to sleep in only if it begins to rain. The next morning the band moves on again in search of food unless there is heavy rainfall throughout the day.

The data from short-term trips (with a range of 4 to 15 days) suggest that as foragers the Ache eat an astounding 3,100 calories per person per day (Hill et al. 1984). (By contrast, active adult Americans consume about 2,700 calories per day.) When the Ache are living in the forest, an average of 56% of their calories come from mammalian meat (ranging from 46% to 66%, depending on the season), with honey making up 18% (range 6-30s) and plants and insects providing an average of 26% (range 15-49%).

In the forest, Ache men spend about 6.7 h/day in subsistence activities (searching, acquiring resources, and processing food) and another 0.6 h/day working on the tools used in subsistence activities. Men also spend about 4.5 h resting, socializing, or in light activities each day (Hill et al. 1985). Women spend about 1.9 h in subsistence activities, 1.9 h moving camp, and about 8 h in light work or childcare (Hurtado et al. 1985). The contrast between the genders may not be surprising in light of the finding that men provide 87% of the energy supplied in the Ache diet and close to 100% of the protein and lipid [fat] consumed.

> ~ Quotation from Hill, K.R. and A. Hurtado: "Hunter-Gatherers of the New World", American Scientist 77 (5):436-443. (1)

Although we can never be 100% sure how the European, Middle Eastern and eventually modern North American African descendants lived, we can be fairly sure that it wouldn't have been a million miles away from our present-day South American cousins.

So with this all this day-to-day wandering, carrying and occasional chasing we can come up with good assumptions about what we were up to thousands of years ago.

The following points seem to be the most important.

- *Hunting was mostly about searching: they did not do hour upon hour of effortful running.*

- *Sometimes, but not every day, they would put in short bursts of hard efforts to catch their prey. (Hill notes that the Ache's day, which he describes so vividly, was harder than any other tribe he visited and that these high levels of effort were not actually the norm.)*

- *The Hiwi and most of the other tribes he studied would usually have a whole day off after high intensity efforts to recover. Rainfall too would sometimes force any tribe to curtail their efforts and probably stay in camp.*

- *The hunter-gatherers movements were highly varied to match the terrain: "...ducking under low branches and vines about once every 20 seconds...and climbing over fallen trees, moving through tangled thorns".*

- *The members frequently had to lift and carry objects on their expeditions and around their camp, so strength was a vital asset.*

- *The terrain under foot was uneven so each footfall would have been much harder than a stroll through the park or a high street.*

- *The women worked a longer day but would have expended less overall energy. Both sexes however left plenty of time for rest, recovery and socializing.*

Ancient movements to modern practice

Just as for modern hunter-gatherers, it's clear that in past millennia we would have had to move a whole lot more. There were no cars to save the shoe leather, no supermarkets with copious food, no 'click of a mouse' ordering online, no easy desk jobs, etc. So life was made up of both sustained, low-effort movements (for example, walking from one hunting ground to another) and the sort of explosive movements necessary to either catch prey or avoid becoming it.

Dr. Kim mentions variation a great deal. Variation in the sort of movements they performed every day; variations in day-to-day energy expenditure (usually in the form of an easy day followed by a harder day); and variation of the total amount of 'exercise' performed by the different tribes he has studied.

89

From this brief insight into the movements of a modern day hunter-gatherer we can learn some broad principles on which we can begin to base our own programme.

Ensure it:

- *is based around easy, sustainable aerobic work (walking is fine).*

- *contains some regular lifting movements to maintain strength and muscle mass (for women as well as men). You don't need to do this every day. Two or three times a week is sufficient.*

- *is built around real human movement patterns, not artificial ones created by machines in a gym. Include plenty of squatting, duck-ing, crawling, jumping, running, throwing, lunging, pulling and lifting.*

- *includes some high-intensity efforts like sprinting, but only a hand-ful of times a week.*

- *alternates easy days and harder days most of the time, taking a day off when you genuinely feel tired or under the weather.*

The lifestyle of modern day hunter-gatherer tribes are an accurate representation of the lives hominids lived for 99.6% of our time on this planet.

A fateful contrast

Please take a moment, if you haven't already, to consider your own day and how it differs. What demands does it generally place upon you? What physical exercise do you get? For many people, in terms of move-ment; it goes something like this:

"Rise, walk a few steps, descend stairs, sit, eat, walk a few steps, five breaths of fresh air, drive, walk a few steps, sit, sit, eat, sit, sit, walk a few steps, sit, stand, walk a few steps, sit, walk, drive, walk a few steps, take five breaths of fresh air, eat, sit, ascend stairs, sleep"

You might be proudly thinking "Well that's not me! I work out!"

If that's the case, you can bet it's a 40-minute period dedicated to exercise. And I'll be prepared to bet it's either a plod on a treadmill or some prolonged form of self-inflicted 'beasting' that pushes you to, and probably beyond, the comfortable limits of your ability.

The tribes in the descriptions above live lives of continual relaxed, varied movement, interspersed with brief, frantic bursts of energy, followed by long periods of relaxation. By contrast, our days are filled with large quantities of sitting, tiny amounts of movement, regular carb-filled meals, and chronic stress. When we look at it like this, it really isn't hard to see how so many of us have gone wrong.

For every little change you can make that takes your experience of life a little closer to that of our hunter-gatherers ancient ancestors, the healthier and the happier you will be.

As mentioned earlier in the book, this really isn't a suggestion of some sort of ancient history re-enactment activity: that you return to the woods, become a hunter-gatherer, throw away your food blender, or try hunting wild pig in Sherwood Forest. However, there are elements of your life that you can change that will serve your hard-wired instincts and improve your life beyond measure.

The advantages of a more natural 'balanced' range of movement, activities and exercise:

*More energy * Better immunity to illness * Lower body fat * Greater muscle mass * More endurance * Better balance * More speed * Greater range of movement and flexibility * Fewer signs of ageing * Less stress * Better moods * Less dependency on drugs * Lowered risk of diabetes*

Mighty big claims, I know!

In the rest of this chapter I will outline how you can easily change your movement habits and patterns to become more like our ancestral patterns – a total workout package. All round fitness shouldn't be about isolating one body part and hitting it intensely to get a single aesthetic result. Your overall vitality is only ever as strong as your weakest link.

We will look at how when exercise is made easy and relaxed (like the Hiwi and the Ache) – and if you adopt movement habits more like our ancestral patterns – you get an unrivaled **total body workout**.

All round fitness shouldn't be about isolating one body part and hitting it intensely to get a single aesthetic result, but an integrated, all over fitness approach that leaves the body balanced, the posture tall and erect, and a strength and grace that no conventional gym workout could ever offer.

But before we move on, I'd like to explain a bit more about my original inspiration for what was to become 'instinctive' fitness: Africa.

Out of Africa

I don't think I would have ever made the connection between so-called 'primitive' peoples and the key to great health and fitness had it not been for my time in Africa training to be a game ranger. By sheer good fortune I was exposed to an effortless, natural formula for fitness and health. My days spent in the bush showed me how fitness could come without fuss and that health runs far deeper than simply not being too fat or too thin.

It seems like an age ago now and yet strangely my memories remain vivid and sharp. I can still hear the relentless, step-after-step crunch of our boots on the dusty shale-strewn trails. We would walk the tough, rugged terrain and I can still taste the arid dryness and recall the glorious relief offered by the merest swig of lukewarm water from a canteen. Those long, relaxed expeditions through the bush were like no walk I have experienced before or since.

Every step presented a new challenge as we were forced to rebalance on uneven ground, scale steep embankments, leap small ravines, scramble up banks, duck under vines and thread our way through rocky, dried up river beds. It was the sheer variety of movement that made a day of walking a challenge; yet it was never boring, repetitive, grueling nor exhausting. It was fully engaging and completely natural.

It felt as if I was leading the life we were born to lead.

For our ancestors, every day was one long camping and hiking trip

Within a few weeks of this, my pasty English legs had turned bronze and I had become conditioned to the myriad of new challenges that had initially so shocked my system. Only a week or two into the course, unless I was required to carry extra weight that day, my legs seemed to move under me as if on autopilot, gracefully finding the perfect foot position and weight distribution for each step. My legs just seemed to flow underneath me without any undue effort or conscious thought.

Slow and steady

More than 90% of our movement was low pace, at a speed at which breathing was unaffected and conversation was easy. Conventional training programmes will tell you this sort of effortless movement is no use to us. "You can't get fit walking," we're all told. "Unless you're pushing hard, breathing hard and 'feeling the burn' you'll never get the results you want" is the oft-repeated myth.

However, from my experience, this is utter rubbish. My days in Africa very rarely contained anything that remotely resembled the sort of punishing session your average club runners put themselves through. According to conventional theory, what I was doing shouldn't be nearly enough to have made a difference – and yet I felt fitter and healthier than I had ever done in my whole life. Even after a 10-hour day on the trail, I rose the next morning raring to go without aches or pain. Through all the apparent hardship, my body felt lighter. *Life* was lighter.

There were a handful of days however that fell outside this leisurely easy pace. On a handful of occasions the 'no-hurry' walking and carrying very much took a back seat.

In particular, the one event that broke the day's gentle pattern was our brush with the buffalo mentioned in Chapter One. This is an event that will remain etched in my mind forever. Rito, our indomitable guide and protector was scouting ahead as usual, seemingly gliding over the ground in his usual way through the dense bush. Our quiet march was brought to an abrupt halt when his slim, muscled torso instantly froze on the path ahead. His arm slowly rose and hand made a fist to signal the need for absolute stillness.

Run like hell

We had practiced this drill often, but this time was for real as we had walked straight into a hide of buffalo entirely hidden by the high grass. (Sneaky little hiders, buffalo.)

The word 'buffalo' probably won't strike up the same feeling of 'danger' as 'lion' or 'rhino' but weighing in at up to a tonne, this mountain of muscle and sinew is extremely bad tempered and unpredictable. The seemingly unglamorous buffalo is indeed a fearsome beast and, as a group, they have been known to take down lions, so a band of gangly humans was no match for them.

Having been previously briefed on the seriousness of such a situation and what to do, my heart was hammering away in my chest and ears. Although every fibre of my being screamed *RRUUUN!* We all followed John our instructor's lead and nervously stood our ground waiting for Rito. We could actually smell the angry buffalo just metres away as they blasted a warning of hot air out of their nostrils as though they might literally explode at us at any second!

None of us petrified trainees panicked as the seconds ticked by, and, at a moment known only to him, Rito slowly retreated backwards into our group, and when he just kept moving right through us and kept going, without instruction we followed his lead and backed away. Once out of immediate sight of the buffalo, Rito took off like a scolded cat to put some distance between them and us.

I didn't know a man in his late 50's could move that fast (in fact I didn't know *I* could move that fast) as we furiously put distance between us and them with more pace and sheer energy than I had ever before experienced – fuelled by the genuine danger and powerful thrill of the encounter.

Because we had escaped a situation, which we knew was potentially lethal (and had been the end of many unwary African natives and quite a few tourists), I felt unbelievably exhilarated. Once at a safe distance our group laughed with relief, excitement and bravado as we exchanged our own personal recollection of what had just happened. Even Rito, for once, appeared slightly ruffled and secretly elated.

I have never before, nor since, felt so totally alive!

For the next few days I was absolutely buzzing. The grass was greener, the sky was bluer and the bush was, er, bushier. This wasn't just some weird personal psychological aberration though: the whole group felt like this. Each and every step we took outside the safe confines of camp was laced with consequence – a new, very real potential for danger: We were living on an exhilarating, natural high.

For some time following 'Buffalogate', it seemed like my newly found indefatigable limbs had discovered yet another gear. Whenever I could find an excuse I would break into a sprint just for the hell of it. I wanted another hit of that energy and euphoria – another stab at that hidden 'turbo boost' button I just couldn't get enough of.

Of course any half-decent physiologist, biologist or psychologist could tell you all about the mysterious 'turbo boost' button we had tapped into – the incredible hormone-boosting power of fight or flight phenomenon.

The body knows far better than we do what it needs at any given time. 99.9% of the time the body is careful to protect itself by keeping well within its own reserves of effort. Recent scientific studies clearly show that it will slow us down with painful warning signals long before the body itself is in any danger of any self-inflicted damage.

When it all gets a bit 'hairy' and the body suspects it's in any real danger of harm, it draws upon a special backup of physical and mental energy, which can save the day in times of emergency.

The whole world goes into slow motion: suddenly heavy things seem light and limbs take on a powerful life of their own. This is the delightful 'fight or flight response.

It took years for me to realise the significance of this fight or flight response, but as a completely natural part of our bodies' repertoire, you can see how it should fit neatly into any truly *instinctive* fitness programme.

Like many other aspects of physical wellbeing, the 'fight or flight' system runs according to the rule of 'use it or lose it', and having let this potent source of hormonal energy out of the box (the neurotransmitters epinephrine and norepinephrine, if you're interested) I didn't want to put it back in.

This fight or flight response was the missing piece of the puzzle for me. It was certainly what my medium pace, medium intensity, medium interest, plodding workouts I had been following at home had been sorely lacking.

Fight or Flight – Bring it on.

This brings us nicely onto the Instinctive Fitness model of exercise which is very much for a modern world, but mimics *all* the daily/weekly physical demands and movements of these healthy, happy, very much 'alive', modern-day hunter-gatherers.

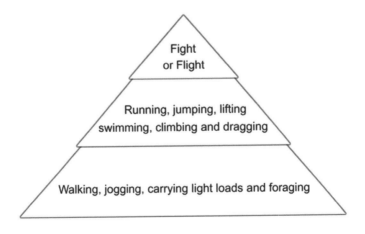

If you really want to get into a 'caveman fit' shape, you're going to need to carry out movements or activities similar to those in the diagram above.

If you do start to adopt a more rounded exercise programme you'll very quickly start to feel healthier, more flexible, more vibrant and more alive. Introducing the Instinctive Fitness model of exercise:

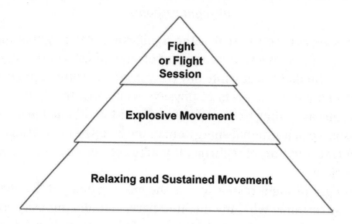

An instinctive approach places its emphasis on just these three core areas.

Compared to the very modern, 'thrash in the gym' style of workout, the Instinctive Fitness model of exercise better serves our genes and instincts. Of course our Stone Age ancestors would never be able to get their heads around the concept of exercise purely for exercise's sake, but this is the model to best replicate their active lifestyles.

The new rules of exercise

There are of course various other elements to consider when it comes to getting 'superfit'. They fall broadly into the following more 'mainstream' categories.

1. *Maximum strength*

2. *Flexibility*

3. *Posture and poise*

4. *Speed, agility and balance*

Let's look at each in turn:

Maximum strength:

Maximum Strength is anyone's maximum instant capacity to move a heavy weight, and a very basic measure of 'maximum strength' is simply the amount you can lift off the ground – once and once only. Now think back to the description of the hunter-gatherers' day, and your own.

How many times are you called upon in your average day to exert your maximum capacity in an instant? Most likely seldom, or never at all – and in all likelihood, the same holds true for the tribesman. Now and again they might have dragged a branch or lifted an animal that was at the absolute edge of their maximum strength, but generally they would have worked safely within their full capacity.

So, in fact, with some further thought, we've established that maximum strength work (category one) isn't much of a day-to-day feature of an ancient lifestyle, so it doesn't need to play a huge role in yours, unless you especially want it to. (You can become an Olympic lifter if you want to – but you don't need to.)

Flexibility

This is something that hunter-gatherers would never have consciously worked at – but then they never had to. They retained the good flexibility that comes with having great natural posture and engaging in natural movement every day. All their movements would have been skillful and mindful; their movement patterns were the result of thousands of hours of subconscious practice.

Today, if working out with a fully-balanced exercise plan, specific flexibility and stretching work should only be strictly necessary in remedial situations when a specific issue is being addressed. For example, a martial artist might need to improve their hip flexibility so that they can kick to head height. For an injured sportsman, this could be regaining a full range of movement in a joint that has recently suffered some damage.

For people who have postural issues and muscle imbalances (most of us), very specific dynamic movements can help rebalance resting muscle length of key muscles, alleviate pain, reduce the likelihood of injury and improve performance. Random, general stretching is unlikely to do this however. The sort of random, haphazard stretching you see going on before most amateur sporting events is likely to do more harm than good.

In general though, if you are active in the widest possible sense, regularly practising complete natural movements and maintaining a good posture through all your activities, you should not require much stretching to maintain good muscle length. Certainly, I don't think our ancestors spent much time stretching, but then they would never have let their level of flexibility get as poor as most of us have. If you do have serious issues a couple of appointments with a human movement specialist may therefore be a very good investment.

> Movement specialists look at your own particular patterns of movement and prescribe a programme for your own, very idiosyncratic body. Check out www.instinctive-fitness.com to find a local approved specialist who will help offset all the unnatural movement patterns and positions you have used habitually for years.

Alternatively if, for example, you have a slightly displaced pelvis (a common issue for many people) you might need a chiropractor to short-cut rehabilitation. In a modern world with modern problems, sometimes the answer is a modern solution – again, check out our website for a good chiropractor.

Posture and poise

There is a whole chapter devoted to this topic, such is its importance. Posture is the very expression of our human nature and how we align with gravity or fight against it defines much of the ease and grace with which we go through life. Our ancestors' posture would have remained good simply by copying the poise and posture that other members of their tribe displayed.

Speed, agility and balance

These are all co-ordination issues. Once you start to exercise and move in a more natural way, the Instinctive Fitness model delivers fantastic speed, agility and balance without needing to specifically practice these in isolation. These last three come naturally when following a more natural or 'functional' fitness plan.

So you can see that for *most* people who don't have a specialised, Olympic ambition, serious physical defect or desire a bodybuilder's muscle mass, the Instinctive Fitness pyramid offers a comparatively painless, easy-to-understand and unbelievably effective route. It's the ideal way to become more active, lose a few pounds and enjoy all the other spin-off benefits we've already covered.

So, let's focus in on what is important

1. *Explosive Movement*

2. *Fight or Flight Sessions*

3. *Relaxed and Sustained Movement*

Here we are focusing on the essential components of a pure thorough-bred human. Trust me, if you can get these qualities nailed down, you will be fitter than pretty much everybody you know. You'll be capable of turning your new found natural fitness abilities to whatever the situation requires – whether that be responding to an emergency or simply leaving every other dad for dead in the Fathers' Race at your kid's school.

Also, while you shouldn't be overly-concerned with appearance, a by-product of the Instinctive Fitness exercise programme is that you'll also end up looking fairly 'ripped'. You'll never look like Stallone or Schwarzenegger in their steroid-fuelled prime, but you've probably got the potential to look a bit like Brad Pitt in *Fight Club* or Linda Hamilton in *Terminator 2*.

If that sounds ridiculous, then remember that I am not suggesting that this sort of change happens overnight. If you are woefully out of shape (I'm thinking – to keep the Hollywood theme going – of the "Nutty Professor" look), then it might take a few years. If you're not as young as you used to be, these changes will take a little longer. But you could certainly get there with enough time and consistency to your efforts.

Even if you don't quite reach these dizzy aesthetic heights (I am not denying differing genetic potentials), if you stick with the right programme you will end up toned, wiry, nimble, fleet-of-foot, powerful for your weight, super-charged with energy and with a whole new vigour about you.

To get the very best results however, you *must* combine any exercise programme with the eating patterns outlined in the coming chapters if you are to get even half-way towards these ideals.

Let's look at these three aspects of true 'instinctive' fitness in turn.

1. Explosive movement

In *Instinctive Fitness* we call any short, sharp, high intensity movement an 'Explosive Movement'. Don't confuse this with your tri-weekly run to exhaustion on your gym's cross-trainer.

Explosive Movement is your body's ability to apply a comparatively high amount of force and to continue to do so over a restricted period of time. Any exertion that extends over this time period results in rapidly getting out of breath, pain and massive performance loss because you'll be using your anaerobic pathway.

Anaerobic what? 'Anaerobic' means 'without oxygen', and when exercising like a demon you'll inevitably very soon notice fatigue and pain in the muscles through lactic acid build up and a quick deterioration in movement quality. Anaerobic exercise is a short, high intensity effort with which your heart and lungs cannot (in the long term) keep up. So in effect, once you are working hard enough to go *anaerobic* you're living on borrowed time and exhaustion is not too far away.

Our ancestors were in this zone when jumping between rocks, climbing trees, running from animals with explosive acceleration and moving heavy branches. They were totally incapable of keeping up any of these feats for an extended period of time, so they didn't even try – but they were capable of pursuing these activities with ease for a constrained period without immediate fatigue or discomfort.

If you are easily fatigued by running fifty yards for a bus, climbing three flights of stairs, using a foot pump, carrying grocery bags, or walking up steep hills, Explosive Movement is an area that might need some serious attention...

Getting into the explosive movement zone

The good news is that this sort of fitness improves quite quickly when you approach it in the right way. Twenty minutes or so of a few brief exertions, two or three times a week, will pay noticeable dividends within a month. (You might not lose much weight in this time, but you will quickly start to avoid fatigue when previously you would have been red-faced and puffing like a choo-choo train.)

The effect of this comparatively high intensity training is to develop your body's ability to supply enough oxygen and glucose to the muscles fast enough. In doing so, additional strength will develop in those muscles. Sometimes with this type of training, muscles grow larger, although this depends on many other factors, especially nutrition. It is more useful as an aid to weight loss and strength building than it is a genuine muscle-building programme.

Undoubtedly, you *will* get considerably stronger, and your physical capacity will grow, but if you measure your biceps every morning you will probably be disappointed; it would be better instead to measure your waistline every week or so.

At this point, having decided that the benefits of this sort of training are definitely for you, you have a few different choices when it comes to implementation.

> Ladies, explosive movements are essential for you as well. The feminine form is just as defined by musculature as the male body, so please, any talk of muscle 'building' absolutely does not mean you will look like a bodybuilder or less lady-like.

To get your body working, shifting a bit of weight and getting your heart rate up doesn't have to involve a running machine, a cross trainer or any other form of equipment. To get the body into the 'explosive movement' zone you have 2 options:

1. *Build this sort of movement into your day with* **Heavy Resistance Tasks** *or*

2. *Commit to an* **Explosive Movement Session** *2 or 3 times a week.*

Explosive movement – Option 1: build heavy resistance tasks into your day

Ideally to take up no more time or effort in your busy day, you would simply do tasks that require this sort of sustained that actually needed doing anyway. Examples of this might be...

- *chopping logs for a fire with an axe rather than using a chainsaw*

- *raking up leaves rather than using a blower*

- *digging a big hole without the aid of a 'mini-digger'*

- *carrying bricks in a wheel barrow*

- *using a sledge hammer rather than a 'breaker'*

- *moving furniture*

Whatever you do – do it with some vigour.

Once people stop moving, it is hard to get started again. Any movement is good at this stage. It shouldn't hurt. Start off nice and easy....

If you are particularly out of shape, perhaps a really thorough vacuuming of the house will get the heart pounding. Include under beds and furniture, dust all the high and low spots to get stretching and bring on a bit of a sweat.

Maybe you could clean the car, weed the garden, cut the grass, or do some painting? Any household chores done with some 'gusto' really will be a good start to get moving again.

If you're a bit fitter, these won't challenge you so much but can still be counted towards your 'Relaxed and Sustained' activities for the week.

Including this sort of activity in your week on a number of occasions will get you reasonably fit and strong. Over time, you can build considerable strength, technique and some reasonable cardiac capacity.

Of course, one advantage of this approach is that if the tasks need doing anyway, it effectively doesn't take up any time at all. Another is that all of these activities involve authentic human movement patterns – unlike the ab-curl machine at the gym, which will only accelerate your transformation into a hunchback.

A disadvantage of relying solely on this approach is that your heart and cardiovascular system won't be worked quite as well as it would be with a more formal workout. (We'll come to this in a bit.)

Who knows? All this log chopping and carrying may have you fancying going the whole hog: moving to a log cabin, growing your own vegetables, raising your own grass-fed livestock, hunting for edible fauna in the woods, living entirely off your own labours... Okay, well maybe not; but somebody might?

Explosive movement – Option 2: commit to two or three explosive movement sessions a week.

For those who live a typical, town-based life of relative ease, hardy, 'outdoorsy' activities of the type described above might be difficult to find.

For those already active and in a reasonable state of fitness, light housework just won't be challenging enough. If you can't easily manufacture the excuse to 'get physical' in your daily tasks, you might need to put some specific time aside to work up a bit of a sweat.

This could be the same identical routine of exercises each day, but ideally you would add variation to maintain interest and encourage progression.

We'll go into a bit more detail later on, but here are the basic principles:

- *Do each exercise until it becomes uncomfortable – then **stop**! You do <u>not</u> need to do any exercise to failure or exhaustion!*

- *Choose movements that are challenging, whole-body, co-ordinated efforts. Bodyweight exercises are ideal for this, but free weights, sandbags, kettlebells and lots of other things (but not gym machines!) are great for variety too. Don't bother trying to isolate muscles.*

- *Arrange your exercises as a circuit, one exercise followed by the next one. (Don't use sets. For our purposes that would be a waste of time and boring) When one area of the body gets a rest, hit that area with the next exercise.*

- *Keep your mind on what you're doing and enjoy the movement for itself.*

- *Incorporate as much variety as possible. Change exercises and make variations within exercises.*

- *Don't let your heart rate drop too much; rest as little as possible between exercises but do be prepared to take a break if your breathing becomes uncomfortably laboured.*

Undoubtedly, many of these basic exercises you'll have come across before but there is a myriad of ways to create the variety of movements that provides the 'hunter-gatherer's edge'. This is done by adding as many seemingly small but vital variations around a natural movement pattern as possible. (Go to www.instinctive-fitness.com for all the information you'll need for a 10-minute home workout)

The six natural movement patterns

1. *Bending, hinging or jumping (to lift something, including yourself, off the ground)*

2. *Pushing (pushing an object away from you, or yourself away from the ground)*

3. *Pulling (pulling an object towards you, or your own bodyweight away from the ground)*

4. *Lunging (forward step with stabilization)*

5. *Twisting (movement of the body on its own axis – the aspect that's missing from almost all conventional gym programmes)*

6. *Gait* (movement with support – stabilization of the core against gravity while allowing movement. e.g. walking, running, crawling or carrying)*

*technically, gait is a highly developed deployment of the other five patterns

Using primal movements like these, the whole body can be worked out in around 10 minutes: muscles, heart and lungs. You can feel great with the kick of adrenaline and endorphins released into the bloodstream that the mind revels in.

At the end of the workout you should feel *more* vital, *more* alive, and *more* ready to go (not searching round for a spot to lie down and die.) This is not because you've suddenly become super-fit; but because you now know exercise *shouldn't* hurt and how to respect your body's current limits.

The following basic five types of exercise exemplify five of these natural movements. The sixth movement (twisting) needs to be built into any selected movement as an essential variation. The exercises below really are the basics and are only a small selection of the many that address each of these six movement patterns.

1. **Press-ups** *[Pressing – for the chest, shoulders, arms, core]*

2. **Squats** *[Bending – for legs and core]*

3. **Pull-ups** *[Pulling – for arms and back]*

4. **Lunges** *[Forward step with stabilisation – for legs and core]*

5. **Crawl** *[Gait – movement with support]*

I'll take just one exercise – the squat – as an example. I'll show you the sort of variations you should use to keep things interesting, effective and challenging.

The squat

This is a vital movement, considered by some to be **the king of exercises**. It creates explosive leg power, lower body stability, increased flexibility, superior endurance and boosted metabolism. It also works the core muscles much harder than you would expect for an exercise that's associated with the lower body.

You know how to do a squat, right?

Well maybe you do and maybe you don't. Most people think they do but actually don't. People who can squat well can do most athletic pursuits well. Those that can't, tend to struggle in most physical endeavours. If you can resist the power of gravity effectively without locking your legs you will excel at sports that involve explosive power from the lower body (which is most of them.) This is not the place to try to teach you proper technique but learning how to do it properly may save you from injury and structural weakness.

On the face of it, the standard repertoire of five exercises above might seem a bit limiting, but with some simple variations the above five core exercises can produce over thousands of possible movements.

Here are some variations of just the squat. You could and should play with these variations; find the ones you most struggle with to make the biggest impact on your fitness and flexibility. The differences may seem on the face of it trivial, but try them and you'll discover the challenge becomes very different with each variation and the muscles that take the strain also differ greatly.

1. ***Foot placement*** *– feet level with each other, shoulder width apart is one of many variations. What about feet wide apart? What about touching? What about one foot forward of the other? This gives you nine alternative foot positions.*

2. ***Foot angle*** *– your feet can point straight ahead, inwards like a pigeon, or outwards like Charlie Chaplin. Multiply this variation by the one above and you've got 27 different varieties of squat.*

3. ***Upper body rotation*** *– who says your upper body has to face the front while you do these? Rotate both your arms to the left or the right as you do these and we're up to 81 variations.*

4. **Arm movement** – *keep your arms well above head (perhaps holding a weight) or drive them down right underneath yourself as reaching for something very low down. (That's 243 if you're still counting)*

But who says both arms have to move the same direction as each other? One arm could drive up while the other drives down – or sideways?

What if we take one leg off the ground and do any of the above variations? (Yes, I've totally lost count now too!)

The point is that the permutations of just this one basic exercise are endless, yet most people who squat will do it just the one way, repeatedly, again and again, until they are totally bored (which probably won't be that long).

Free movement resources

On the IF website at *www.instinctive-fitness.com* there are many videos/ pictures showing many Explosive Movement exercises – even simple ones for those who might initially struggle to get started. And remember, these aren't just for beginners either – each and every essential movement pattern can be made scalable – both easier and harder, depending on your current level of fitness.

What's crucial to this approach is that it must never *ever* hurt. If this isn't your experience of this sort of exercise – you're doing it wrong. You don't need to push yourself beyond the natural boundaries that your body lays down for you. Your body knows how much exercise it needs to progress and will try to protect you by reducing your enjoyment of the experience.

Stay within your body's pain boundaries and enjoy the experience – so you'll come back and enjoy it again tomorrow.

When exercise hurts, one part of the mind remembers the experience and finds all sorts of excuses not to participate in this sort of ritual ever again. This is when it becomes difficult to find the motivation to work out. When the mind behaves like this, it is throwing the baby out with the bath water, but you have spent time conditioning it to believe that exercise must be effortful and uncomfortable – so you can hardly blame it for adding two and two in this way.

"Exercise is labour without weariness."
Samuel Johnson

A challenge for you

If you want a real challenge, instead of seeing how knackered you can feel at the end of an activity or workout, see if you can complete a workout while only breathing deeply through your nose. With practise it *is* possible and ensures that you never leave the boundaries within which your body will prosper, enjoy and thank you for.

Enjoy yourself

Follow your interest, your heart and your feelings. If you hate an exercise, don't do it. If a movement hurts, don't do it. If you feel seriously uncomfortable on the tenth repetition, just do seven – or whatever feels comfortable. When it stops being interesting and challenging and just seems like a slog, STOP!

Remember that if you are "scheduled" to complete a session but you feel under the weather or poorly-recovered from a previous session, just rest that day and restart your routine when you feel raring to go again.

If your enthusiasm is flagging, it could be that your body actually needs more rest and is trying to secure it for you by reducing your enthusiasm. If your body needs rest, it'll let you know one way or another. There's no need for heroics. Leave your 'whatever-it-takes' Rambo mentality for real emergencies.

Mix it up – make it fun

If you feel you're getting stale, mix it up a bit. You could try new variations of an exercise; new exercises entirely; a change of venue (get outside); or find something different to lift than your own bodyweight. (What about a tractor wheel, a sandbag or a rock?)

With all of these exercises, focus on form, as if you were being assessed for grace rather than strength endurance. Don't kick yourself if you don't do each movement well yet. Treat each movement as *practise*, instead of just a task or exercise.

Try to do movement and exercises that fit into all of the 6 Natural Movement Patterns listed above. Don't, for example, just focus on pull-ups because you're good at them.

2. Fight or flight sessions

People 'in training' typically push themselves 'quite hard', 'quite a lot'. They do the same thing each week but they either get increasingly tired over time (without enough recovery time) or they progress little as their sessions never raise the bar of their maximal efforts. This is what I used to do before I saw the light and it's a recipe for failure – as my belly would attest.

If you perform the above movements regularly or organise your life so that plenty of resistance tasks are built into it, you will already be on the way to improving your aerobic capacity (that is, the ability of the heart and lungs to provide your muscles with the oxygen and fuel that they require).

However, if you think back to the description of the modern day hunter-gatherer tribes' brief but energetic hunt, or the mad dash away from the buffalo herd during my days in the African bush, there's another form of fitness we've left unexamined so far: Fight or Flight.

Of course back in Paleolithic times, this adrenalin-fuelled, furious, life or death activity might only happened irregularly. Some weeks they might have had to 'run for their lives' twice a day, and other weeks not at all, but we can be sure any hunter-gatherer wouldn't have gone too long without a brief, 100%, 'peddle to the metal' effort.

This all-out, frantic activity is the crucial point most people miss when designing a training programme, so it's perhaps the biggest secret there is. Most people struggle to get the results they're looking for because their routine is very predictable – 60-70% effort – and they never push the dial right up to ten.

Predictable routine training produces predictably average results

Middle ground to nowheresville

Remember that one of our ten, hard-wired, human instincts is to be as lazy as possible. Except when sudden, dire, adrenalin-filled situation occurred, we would have walked to our destination in an unhurried fashion, and sprinted very occasionally when the situation demanded it.

Go to a running club if you're unconvinced. You won't see much lean muscle mass there. Instead you'll see surprisingly chubby people whose fat tissue has managed to survive all those miles, people with emaciated frames (the beanpoles), or people who have both issues going on (the 'skinny-fat'). You won't see anyone who looks like a sprinter, with noticeably defined muscle, spontaneous power and low body-fat.

This is why, unless you're doing a fight or flight session, training should *always* be easy, even when you're doing explosive movement sessions or working around the house. Don't grind yourself into the ground over the course of weeks.

It's ironic that the marathon event was inspired by the fortunes of its first runner, the Greek Pheidippides, who collapsed and died after completing his feat of endurance. This is an event that people now take up for 'health reasons' and yet the evidence suggests quite the opposite. Regular distance racers suffer depressed immune systems and enjoy a low level of health.

A recent study from the University of Melbourne showed that high-effort endurance activities could lead to scarring of the right ventricle (heart chamber), increasing the risk of health complications. The researchers followed 40 marathon runners and discovered that all of the runners suffered from decreased function of the right ventricle for about a week after the race; in five of them the damage to their heart appeared to be permanent.[1]

The occasional long distance event is fine if you fancy taking part, but take it easy and don't log hundreds of tough miles in preparation for it. In fact, choose an event that is a surprise to your body but doesn't overly tax it. Just enjoy it without worrying about your finishing position. Then allow for plenty of recovery time.

'Distance racing' – whether running, cycling, swimming or triathlon – is fine under these conditions but, if fitness is your goal, entirely optional. All you'll achieve by flogging yourself is to add a lot of stress to your life, and probably quite a lot of muscle wastage.

However, there is one bout of the training that is more exciting, more fun, more rewarding than any other and really gets me and my clients into amazing shape: fight or flight.

For these explosively exciting sessions, all prohibitions about never pushing yourself get screwed up and lobbed out the window.

For just a few glorious moments you get to exert maximal efforts, as if your life depended on it. (One day it might!) This high intensity approach should leave you feeling exhilarated and re-invigorated. But here's the thing: it should all be done in a very small window of time. Just a few minutes including recovery time is ideal.

Because each burst of movement is so short it's not, psychologically speaking, that hard at all. You should be able to recover from these efforts pretty quickly – not because you've held back, but because your efforts didn't last very long.

Our Fight or Flight training approach was inspired by a Japanese researcher called **Nishimura Tabata** who developed what he called the IE1 Protocol. (Catchy title, huh?)

This groundbreaking scientist showed that short, high-intensity bursts of movement (four minutes a day, four times a week) could get participants as fit as a control group of trained athletes who logged sessions *more than five times longer.*[2] By the end of the study the former group had a higher VO2 Max (peak oxygen uptake) and, unlike the control group, has also improved their aerobic capacity.

The benefits are indisputable. HIIT (High Intensity Interval Training) has been shown to improve maximal oxygen consumption and, more recently, to improve insulin action and blood-glucose levels.

"Your body knows best"

With Instinctive Fitness we've taken Tabata's principles one-step further by avoiding prescriptive formulas completely and just listening closely to the body. No longer will you need a personal trainer to tell you exactly how long your intervals should be or how much recovery time you are allowed. Instead you'll learn to rely on your own instinct for what's best for you.

It has been shown in studies that the human brain protects the body by sending messages (in the form of pain) telling it to back away from using its full capacity long before it reaches a dangerous level of exertion. Dire emergencies are a notable exception to this rule however. When these happen, hormones flood the body allowing one-off 'superhuman' performances from ordinary, untrained individuals that go down in urban legend: people lifting heavy vehicles off crash victims – that sort of thing.

In the IF system of high intensity training, we make use of this natural protective mechanism to greatly reduce the chance of stress, injury and failure. We prefer to listen and respond appropriately to pain rather than to push through it.

The information and feedback your own body provides is 100% accurate, totally natural and offers a safe method for anyone to safely reach their personal optimal training intensity, without any pain and without ever over-stressing themselves.

Here's how we do it:

The Instinctive Fitness 'fight or flight' protocol

1. *Choose a method of whole-body movement like running, biking, swimming, free-weight squatting or rowing. (Sprinting on the spot is a great option for beginners or those short on equipment or space.)*

2. *Perform this movement at your absolute top speed until your body tells you to slow down. This may be in the form of a noticeable performance drop off, or through other physical signs such as painful, laboured breathing, a stitch, other signs of physical discomfort, or just a disinclination to continue.*

3. *The very moment you feel your body is telling you to back off: BACK OFF! Drop your movements down to a very gentle aerobic level (perhaps 10% of your previous effort).*

4. *Maintain this level until your body returns to a comfortable, steady level and tells you it's ready to go again.*

5. *Repeat the cycle until your body is unable to return to a steady, comfortable level. If you're not raring to go flat out again **within three minutes***: STOP!

This whole session is likely to be over in just a few minutes. Nevertheless, according to all the research on HIIT, this represents a credible and effective method for anyone, no matter what their current fitness level or how hectic their schedule, to stave off the spectre of Type-2 diabetes and obesity.

The great thing about this very personal approach is that it grows with you. You will never have to make any decisions about progression, or need to consciously push any harder with each new session. The feedback your own body gives will automatically let you push just that little bit further without trying, minimising the risk of over-exertion or injury.

Before a session like this you'll probably want to warm up a little first. We'll cover this in greater depth later in the book, but suffice to say that all you really need to do is to practise the movements that you are about to perform in a less intense manner. If you are going to sprint, for example, you might first run 30m, then 50m, then 70m, getting up to a higher speed each time.

If you are coming into this session after hours of sitting down, it might be best if you did some walking or general movements first, as cold muscles can be quite tight and prone to injury if suddenly stressed. If you are totally unfit you should take things steady, running at perhaps only 80% of your top speed for the first few sessions.

This session could all be done in 5-10 minutes (including the warm-up time). If you are aiming to burn fat, then doing this sort of thing on an empty stomach (maybe first thing in the morning) is an amazing short cut to fat loss.

Do this once or twice a week instead of breakfast and you're onto a secret that has been entirely overlooked by mainstream conventional wisdom. If you're not already doing something like this, add it to your programme and watch excess flab melt away and your fitness levels soar.

Living on the edge

If you really need to 'feel the burn' during your fight or flight training, that's fine – but please bear in mind that, from an evolutionary point of view, our ancestors would never have dreamed of deliberately leaving themselves vulnerable to predators by pushing through to total exhaustion.

If you absolutely can't help yourself, and really *must* push your personal limits and feel some pain – only do so for a **maximum of 20-30 seconds**. Pushed beyond this, future performances will not necessarily be the better, and you are certainly compromising your health and immune system.

Sprint like a lion's after you

Remember when you were a kid and you sprinted around the playground for probably no reason, perhaps chasing a football and a whole host of other games were as natural as reaching for the TV remote is now? Remember the thrill and the excitement of games such as 'kick the can' or even good old-fashioned 'chase'?

If you haven't run at full pelt for a long, long time, and when you did give it bash, it felt awkward and your legs just didn't have the zap in them they used too, you'll like this next section.

Sprinting as hard as you can is perhaps one of life's extreme physical pleasures: the feeling of skimming across the ground with (when done in the spirit of play) a lightness and an agility perhaps long since considered consigned to the history books.

Running for short distances is not only great fun, but has a whole heap of health benefits:

1. *Sprinting reduces body fat and reduces insulin sensitivity. (Ever heard of a fat, diabetic sprinter?)*

2. *Sprinting requires maximal recruitment of muscle, so it targets fast twitch muscle fibres much better than slower training. Fast-twitch fibres are thicker than slow twitch fibres, and it is fast twitch fibres that grow in size when activated by the right training.*

3. *Sprinting naturally increases Human Growth Hormone (HGH). HGH increases muscle mass; thickens and adds flexibility to the skin; enhances the immune system; promotes weight loss through fat redistribution and loss; and increases stamina.*

4. *Sprinting strengthens your cardiovascular system with brief bursts of high intensity. Depending on the recovery time you allow yourself, you can work your cardiovascular system more intensely (short recoveries, Tabata style) or concentrate on power, speed and strength (using longer recoveries).*

5. *Sprint workouts are short and a lot more fun than long, boring cardio workouts.*

Go on, find any old excuse – race your children, kick and chase a ball – anything you can think of to re-ignite that urge to run you felt naturally as a child.

Fasted exercise

Conventional wisdom will recommend that you should always fuel up before exercise, and always eat three meals a day – plus snacks. However a moment's thought will make it abundantly clear that we didn't evolve with an entirely consistent calorie supply. Our intake of calories would have been irregular and would have depended on our hunting skill and foraging luck.

Sometimes our ancestors would have gone to bed hungry having tried and failed to find food during the day. Days would often have begun without food, and further 'exercise' would be required again before they were likely to acquire any. In other words, if you're serious about copying our ancestral lifestyle patterns (and serious about fat-loss and health), when you are hungry you should sometimes choose to exercise instead!

Please note that I am not asking you to reduce your calorie intake over anything more than 12 hours, or to do this day after day, as most 'diets' require. To do so, is unnecessary, psychologically tough, and usually backfires. Few can stick with it – but those who do find that much of their reduced weight is not actually fat loss but the disappearance of lean muscle tissue. Almost all later return to their previous weight or heavier, but at a higher percentage body-fat and a lower percentage of muscle. Don't do it.

Our health can no longer afford for us to reactively eat every single time we feel the faintest pangs of hunger, nor to continually deprive ourselves of the nutrients and calories our bodies need. A little rational thought and a tiny dose of discipline allows us to reestablish eating patterns that forged the health and vitality of our ancestors.

All I ask is that you consider – either tactically or for convenience – skipping a meal or two each week. I'll give you details on how to do this later in the book.

Review

Let's see what we've got so far:

1. **Explosive movements** – *Daily resistance tasks such wood chopping or a circuit routine that maintains/builds muscle mass, strength, stamina and high-end aerobic capacity. (10-30 minutes, 2 or 3 times a week)*

2. **A 'fight or flight' session** – *perhaps on a fasted stomach, for weight loss, speed, hormone and immune system optimisation and anaerobic capacity. (15 minutes, maximum, including warm up – 1 or 2 times a week at the most)*

Finally, we need to address the bedrock of the instinctive approach to exercise:

3. Relaxed and sustained movement

Relaxing and sustained movements are essentially a solid quantity of low-level, low-intensity movements. Our ancestors varied between being well rested and performing a considerable amount of low-key movement. A typical estimation by anthropologists is that they covered 7-12 miles a day. Some days they might not have gone very far at all if food stocks were high, but on other days they might cover as many as the full 12 miles.

In the modern age, many of us will struggle to add this sort of level of time commitment into our day. Luckily it's not really needed. Most of the benefits associated with low-level aerobic work can be enjoyed with considerably less time investment. However to be Caveman fit, there is no getting away from doing *some*.

At an absolute minimum you should be looking at three to five hours a week of gentle, sustainable movement. With this you will still accrue 70% of the benefits of being mobile for up to ten times longer. You will certainly avoid the massive risks that have been identified with being completely sedentary.

If you cannot be gently active for more than three hours (out of the 168) in your week, consider that the threat of the sedentary lifestyle has been identified as a continued threat even to those who work out regularly if the rest of their time is divided between being seated and being in bed.

Logging three to five hours of activity might not be as tough as you think. First, sport counts and it's easy to keep up the time if it's fun. If you play a round or two of golf a week, you're covered. If you play tennis twice a week, you'll be most of the way there (same for squash, badminton, etc). I recommend you play these sports just for fun and don't worry about pushing yourself hard; just enjoy the game and enjoy the process.

If sport isn't your thing then just walk (which is ideal), or cycle or swim slowly. Maybe take a couple of dance lessons (almost any dancing is fine – even if it's just on the Wii). Perhaps get a dog to walk – or borrow one. Or start walking to work. Or walk to the shops and carry your shopping back. (Wow... now that's starting to sound very instinctive, isn't it? Nothing artificial about that at all as long as you can pretend you don't have a car!)

If you've added resistance tasks into your day, they also count towards fulfilling this requirement, as long as your body has recovered from them by the next day.

Anything that gets you moving in any way, shape or form is fine; the point is to try to get at least three hours a week where you're not sitting around doing nothing (or working, watching TV or whatever).

Other physical training

The workout programme outlined above is far from the only way to achieve any fitness goals, and there are plenty of other things you can do instead.

If in doubt, refer back to our ancient model of fitness and see where any other suggestions align, if at all, with the life of a typical hunter-gatherer.

From the description of the Ache and Hiwi's days earlier, you'll have noticed that everything they do involved moving themselves and natural objects around the landscape, so it makes perfect sense to try to keep as close to this model as possible.

Therefore walking is better than cycling and using your own body-weight is better than using any sort of a machine as resistance. Most of the time you should be reconnecting with these natural movement patterns, but an occasional bike or rowing machine workout is harmless enough. The need for variety to maintain interest and include as many natural movement patterns in a programme as possible can't be stressed enough.

Get some toys

One deviation from body-weight work you might want to make at some point, especially for men, is to make an investment in a barbell and a set of free weights. This allows a greater degree of strength to be maintained and more muscle growth than using bodyweight alone. A heavy sandbag would make a good alternative too, as would a kettlebell or a 'sloshball'. However, I would consider these unnecessary for most people until they can attain some basic benchmarks – for men, say 40 press-ups, 12 pull-ups and 50 deep squats.

For women, as a rule of thumb it's half of this, but as mentioned earlier, please don't fear a muscly body just because you've lifted a few weights. Unless you start going seriously heavy on the iron, the carbs and protein shakes you will not lose your femininity. Check out Olympic gold medalist in the heptathlon, Jessica Ennis. Does she look masculine?

In a perfect world, all the movements (the squat, press, crawl, etc) would just be part of a spontaneous expression of life – as it was for our forest-dwelling antecedents. For example, a walk of a good length with some light jogging, followed by quick sprints, finished off with a variety of lifting and carrying activity simulates the pressures of a hunter-gatherer's day more realistically than doing all these things separately, on different days.

At www.instinctive-fitness.com we have material that supports a more creative, spontaneous approach to workouts.

Warm up

With that point in mind, warming up before sessions is probably a good idea, but there is an embarrassing deficit of evidence to back-up the claim that stretching reduces the likelihood of injury.

I serious doubt whether our Paleo cousins (or any other animal) stretched out their calves before running from a sabre toothed tiger...

If you *are* going to stretch before workouts, you need to know that exercise science has moved on from the days when static (stationary) stretches were recommended. It is almost universally accepted now that dynamic (moving) movements are preferable.

You wouldn't guess this though if you watch the warm-up at many grass-level sports clubs. Here you'll still see players trying to balance on one foot, pulling the other up behind their thigh in an attempt to give it a good pre-workout 'stretch'. This has been shown to tire the muscles unnecessarily and reduce coordination and performance.

If there is still any case to be made for static, yoga-like exercise, then it is post-workout or between workouts; never before.

The best way to warm up is to go through the same movements that you will be making in the main phase of the warm-up, albeit more slowly, with less weight and with fewer repetitions. This will prepare the mind, warm the muscles, increase the range of movement and raise the pulse for the exertion that is to follow.

Going hardcore

If you have completely bought into this analysis of the hunter-gatherer's day and the need to have an exercise plan (and indeed a lifestyle) that resembles it, then you may be wondering if there isn't value in constructing a workout that even more closely resembles the challenges that hunter-gatherers faced every day. Could you not be chasing, twisting, jumping, crawling, carrying, throwing, climbing, balancing and maybe even fighting?

The answer is an unequivocal and resounding 'Yes!' The earlier 'exercises' are only approximations of these very same movements, but they are not quite the same thing as doing them for real. If you can enact – with the spirit of playfulness, exploration and maybe imagination – scenarios where you feel great about doing all these movements, you can throw away all prescriptive exercise forever.

You can do all these movements anywhere, given a bit of space and a few bits of basic equipment, but you might also wonder if it would not be better to actually train in the forest or other wild, natural environment using logs, fallen trees, rocks, branches and tree stumps as our training equipment?

Again, yes! For those for whom the 'call of the wild' beckons, there is a whole new level of contact with our human roots to be gained from applying yourself in this way. This sort of training (or more accurately, self-development) is growing increasingly popular and it's almost single-handedly down to the efforts of an inspiring Frenchman called Erwan Le Corre. His YouTube video, 'The Workout that Time Forgot,' might be the most inspirational training montage ever filmed. (See **www.movnat.com**)

MovNat training brings people together to run, jump, climb, balance, jump, swim, lift, carry, and even fight. They concentrate on these natural movements in all of their training and it's considered by its adherents to be the most functional form of training available.

I have taken many clients into the forest to train and they love it. We've lifted logs, carried rocks, climbed boulders, crawled up slopes, pulled ourselves up and onto branches, jumped streams – and had some sensational sessions.

Is all this essential? No. Is it preferable? Maybe. The movement patterns are certainly more random and diverse, which has to be good; but it's an individual thing. Many people have lost the ability to express themselves spontaneously in this way. It would need a whole other book to put most people on track with this way of being, thinking and moving. As far as training environment is concerned, there are certainly great benefits to outdoor exercise – but we don't all have to get right back to nature in all its mucky glory to get the most of the benefits available to us.

Truth be known, I would personally choose to be out in the elements, surrounded by nature every day (except in the very foulest of weathers), but it takes a greater leap of faith for many to adopt this approach in conservative, middle England. Indeed I have some clients who want to be trained in their own living rooms, but we will still always focus on natural human movements. For practicality's sake and to keep this book realistic for my typical reader I would say this:

Get moving wherever is convenient and feels right for you. Find a range of activities that fit into the categories of Fight or Flight, Explosive Movement and Relaxed and Sustained Movement. Ensure most of them are based around natural human movement – and lastly – enjoy them.

Final thought for the chapter

I hope this chapter has given you a refreshing perspective on what exercise can do for us, how we should do it and some inspiration to start something new. I also hope it has given you a viable new alternative to the joyless, stuffy, lycra-clad, machine dominated, conventional gym.

The exercise philosophy and routines outlined genuinely represent a new impetus that people can believe in and start practicing in their home today, right now even... and that was always my aim when I started this project.

Go on, give it a try: commit to a week of the real easy stuff. Make sure it never hurts and please let me know how you get on.

Key chapter points:

- *Movement is life: looking to improve the quantity and quality of our movement has to be a central axiom of any approach to a better and longer life.*

- *Our bodies expect natural movement (not gym movement), so make your movements as much like our ancestors as possible.*

- *Concentrate on Explosive Movement, short Fight or Flight sessions and Relaxed, Sustained Movement.*

- *Build Explosive Movement into your day or start a regular routine. Skip any extended cardio work (running, rowing etc) that leaves you breathing heavily for more than 15 minutes.*

- *Be sure to include 3-5 hours of low-key aerobic movement into your week. Walking is fine, or any low-stress sport.*

- *Combine your exercise (especially Fight or Flight) with a missed meal for amazing fat-burning results.*

References:

1. La Gerche A, et al "Exercise-induced right ventricular dysfunction and structural remodelling in endurance athletes" Europena Heart Journal 2011; DOI: 10.1093/eurheartj/ehr397.

2. Tabata I, Nishimura K, Kouzaki M, et al. (1996) "Effects of moderate-intensity endurance and high-intensity intermittent training on anaerobic capacity and VO2max". Med Sci Sports Exerc 28(10): 1327–30.

CHAPTER SEVEN

Natural Posture

"If one's posture is upright, one has no need to fear a crooked shadow"
- Unknown

The collapse of modern society

The movements and eating patterns described in the previous chapters are all essential elements, but for maximum performance and comfortable longevity, there's something else we must consider. Our early ancestors had the advantage of a posture free from the deformities caused by modern comforts, their bodies still working just how evolution intended.

I know good posture is not something that gets talked about much anymore, and you may now be thinking I'm going in a stiff and starchy direction here, but you'll soon find out that good posture is the essential foundation upon which the 'Instinctive' approach is built.

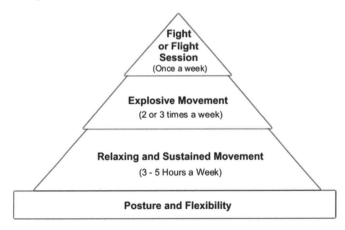

Visualise one of those great big tower cranes you see looming over a city skyline. Picture its girder framework standing straight and strong, lifting heavy loads effortlessly and in great safety. Now imagine you're standing at the bottom watching it at work when you notice its girder framework is badly twisted and bent. There's a great bow in its central pillar warping the whole structure. Someone has even offset the cab right at the top in a vain attempt to keep it balanced. You're shocked to hear it creak and groan alarmingly when it lifts a heavy load. How safe do you feel standing there? Fancy a trip up to the cab?

Spinal collapse

Most individuals suffer – knowingly or not – from a collapse in their spinal structure. In most people, the spine, which should be the foundation of our life-long fight against gravity, is nowhere near the shape it evolved to be. In the western, developed world there are very few exceptions to this. Spinal collapse is one of the most debilitating conditions affecting our society today and this leads to a great number of issues:

- *Pain (in the back, or 'referred pain' to the knees, hips and other areas)*
- *Reduced health (our internal organs become damaged through compression)*
- *Fatigue and reduced zest for life*
- *Reduced mobility, muscle imbalances and flexibility problems*
- *Lack of co-ordination, efficiency and reduced sporting performance (It's no coincidence that the best athletes are those who frequently exhibit the very best spinal health and postures: look at Kenyan distance runners or Jamaican sprinters.)*
- *A bent, twisted, unattractive look*

Before we look at what can be done about this, let's see if we can pin down exactly what we're talking about. The most obvious way you become aware that your spine is out of kilter is that your back hurts – it really is that simple. We've come to accept back pain as a normal fact of life, but it shouldn't be. If it does hurt, even periodically, you're not alone and you are sharing the experience of 95% of the developed world.

In contrast, it is interesting to note that, even without medical care, drugs and therapists, large swathes of the developing world have less than five percent occurrences of back pain, even when engaged in a lifetime of heavy labour. There are women in Africa and Asia who spend up to 10 hours a day working bent over in paddy fields who report no difficulties with maintaining this position and continue to work in this way into old age. A typical westerner could not work for more than a couple of hours before their bent spine would be racked with pain...

If you have back pain – usually lower-back pain – you experience first-hand the effects of this almost universal western malaise. Others might only rarely suffer back pain and not notice the more insidious effects of poor posture. Even if you believe you're in good health, you will find that there will clues that you are in less than good alignment.

Consider the following:

1. *Do you find it tiring standing for longer periods of time?*

2. *Do you find yourself slumping lower in your chair as time passes?*

3. *Do you find that you store tension in your shoulders? Maybe you have a tension 'knot' between your neck and your shoulders?*

4. *Do you find yourself off balance when you reach for things?*

5. *Do your knees hurt or click when they bend? Do your heels come off the floor when you squat onto your haunches?*

6. *Does it feel like your head tries to disappear into your neck when you bend over? Can you keep your back straight when bending forward from the hips (like the women who work in the fields I mentioned earlier)? Or does your upper body curl over like a large letter 'C'?*

7. *Hold your arms extended above your head in front of a mirror. Now squat until your knees are parallel. Notice:*

   a) *Do your knees move out smoothly over the second toes of each foot as they should, or do they pitch inwards (knock-kneed)?*

   b) *Do your arms stay vertically above your head, or are you forced to lower them as you squat?*

   c) *If you can keep your arms vertical, can you still squat fully and comfortably without arching your mid-back?*

8. *Do you have difficulties turning your head fully (90 degrees) to the left or right without also moving either shoulder?*

Testing by appearances

With practise you can look at someone and see if they hold themselves in good alignment. We can think of the different segments of our body as building blocks. Like any sort of structure (imagine a stack of cardboard boxes in a warehouse), it only has real integrity when each block is balanced properly over the others. If one segment is out of kilter, all the rest must be too in order to maintain any sort of balance. Like building bricks, any deviance from the perfect stack results in instability and structural weakness. In the case of our bodies, we require additional energy and tension in the muscles to remain upright. It also results in an unpleasing asymmetry.

How to check your posture

Take a photo of yourself in profile (use a mirror if necessary) wearing only your underclothes. Open it up in a programme like Photoshop, or just print it so you can draw on it. Now draw a plumb line straight upward (90° perpendicular to the floor, parallel with any walls) from your heels, straight through whatever is vertically above it.

If you are in good alignment, the line should pass through the ankle, knee, hipbone, shoulder and ear like the left hand figure, opposite. The central figure has rotated her pelvis forwards too far and then pulled her shoulders and chest up. The figure on the right has gone the other way; she has pushed pelvis backwards too far, rounded her shoulders, pushed her head forward, and now stands in a slump.

If you stand like the figure on the left, congratulations! You are one of the few people I know who has managed to maintain good alignment and pose, even after the end of childhood. You are a rare exception indeed. Most people in the UK, Europe and North America (i.e. most of those living in the developed world) will fail this test.

What is 'correct posture'?

Many people who are concerned or proud of their posture make an effort to correct it. Typically, they find themselves standing or sitting slumped over and then resolve to brace themselves 'upright'. Many people have been making this 'correction' movement for so long they are no longer aware that they spend all day hauling themselves upright.

The military teaches its recruits to force themselves into 'good posture' from day one. Unfortunately these efforts are all based around a false premise: that additional effort can overcome the underlying problem of malcoordination.

There is no single, correct, fixed position for the human body to assume, but there will always be some recognisably 'right' positions under certain fixed conditions.

One such condition is standing still. If you can do this well, without fixing yourself into that position, you will instantly and instinctively make the minimum adjustments needed to cope with additional challenges, such as bending, jumping or walking.

As the old adage says, we must 'learn to walk before we run'; in the

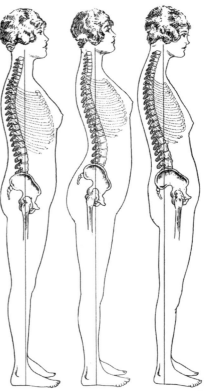

same way we must learn to stand before we can walk – there is a natural hierarchy to these things. Learning to stand well, sit well, and even lie well is essential if your body is to retain or regain the natural symmetry that will keep you pain free, healthy, efficient and relaxed.

Maybe you think you have these qualities already? Maybe people have told you that you have 'great posture' or you just don't ever get back pain, hip pain, shoulder ache – or any of these things I've listed?

So how is your posture?

Take another look at your whole-body profile shot in Photoshop (the one with your plumb line).

Look for these things:

Do any of the key markers I listed above fall out of line with that plumb line? If they do – even just one of them – there are things you need to work on. Even if you think all those markers line up down the plumb-line, it's possible that you are using far too much effort to hold yourself in a fixed, immobile position.

The most likely thing you will see is that your hips are pushed well forward of the marker line. If that's the case, it's almost certain that your head will be too. You will experience 'Forward Head Syndrome' in almost every movement.

Here is a young teenager whose spine is already clearly bent out of shape by gravity:

"Forward head syndrome"

Believe it or not, this is actually the American boy-singer and teenage 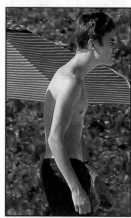 heartthrob, Justin Bieber. (You may not have heard of him if you're not female, into music and about 12 – but if this posture becomes habitual, he won't keep his millions of screaming fans for long.) What kind of example is this icon of teenage vitality unintentionally setting for our youth?

If you think this applies to you, you will probably try to fix the problem by holding your head in a different manner. Don't. You will just add another layer of tension over the layers you already carry. Your head (your uppermost balance block) is misplaced because the blocks underneath it are misplaced too. Your head needs to go where it is at present because, without adding yet more tension, you will just fall over if it goes elsewhere – and that would look even sillier!

> Your head is probably leaning forward to counterbalance your back... which is too far behind the plumb line... because your pelvis is too far in front of the plumb line... because ... oh, you get the idea.

Consider now why so many of us bent out of shape like this. Why are so many of us being sentenced to an old age where we can only shuffle along looking at the ground?

We have already looked at one obvious reason for this malady: a sedentary existence. The term has two meanings, both of which are applicable. We often use the term to denote a life without much movement. This is certainly a contributing factor in this epidemic of badly-stacked people. In effect, lack of movement leads to inflexibility and weakness, whereas flexibility and strength are required to align well.

Get off your backside!

The other sense in which we are sedentary is the more literal interpretation: *we sit, sit, sit, and sit.* Here it's not just the inherent lack of movement that is a problem; it's the actual process of sitting itself that's so harmful to us.

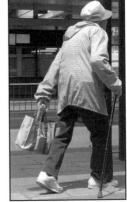

Sitting is a modern aberration. In fact, the majority of the world doesn't 'sit' at all and doesn't want to. If you visit Africa or Asia, you will find most people opt naturally for an alternative resting position: the squat.

And it's not actually just the less developed nations that consider sitting on chairs to be an anathema. Consider the Japanese, an affluent, sophisticated country. They continue to prefer to kneel at low tables rather than to place their (usually well-aligned) spines on chairs. As in the rest of Africa and Asia, this traditional position is part of an ancient culture and has remained unchanged for thousands of years.

In the western world – yet again – things are different. As soon as chairs were invented, they were seized upon as a form of status symbol. To be raised off the ground (on a throne, for example, to take the ultimate symbol of power) was to be exalted over those that sat beneath you.

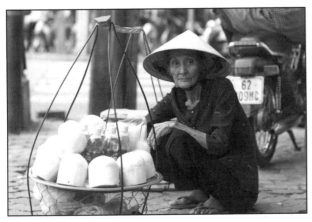

For people from countries that haven't yet fallen for the charms of the armchair and who are well practiced in squatting from childhood through their whole lives, this position isn't hard at all. They find it easy and restful – a position they can sit in for hours.

127

The issue with chairs is that they need a high level of physical aware-ness to be used properly without slow, almost unnoticeable, damage to your posture, spine and balance. Over time, the poor use of chairs re-duces your ability not only to sit properly, but to stand properly, walk properly, and even to lie down beneficially to rest.

Interestingly, this hasn't always been the case. You might expect me to tell you that the rot set in from the very first moment a human sat on a chair, but you'd be wrong.

It seems that chairs have only been as harmful as they are for about 70 to 90 years. In order for the full harmful effects of hours a day in a chair to be felt, something else is needed too: diminished kinesthetic awareness (our sense of what it feels like to be in good alignment).

When this becomes impaired (through factors we'll look at soon) the presence of chairs in our lives seriously exacerbates any issues in a vicious circle that lowers our physical capacity considerably. We have issues – so we sit badly – so the issues worsen – so we sit worse... And so the cycle continues.

As I've suggested, our diminished kinesthetic awareness dates back not to the advent of agriculture, as you might expect me to say, but only less than a century. I suspect that the alignment of hunter-gatherers was better than most of those who worked in fields; however, the biggest change occurred only in the 1920s.

As many of you will know, until recently a part of every young lady's education was deportment lessons. This acknowledges the importance given by society at this time to the quality of standing well and mov-ing well. We used to talk about people moving with 'grace and poise' – terms that are generally out of favour today. Perhaps they sound a bit old-fashioned or elitist to us?

Babies and very young children can sit in a reasonably well-designed chair pretty well. And so can about 1 in 300 adults. But most people can't – and they suffer badly for that fact

---

Not all of the training given to young people and the practice they sustained in later life was of a first class nature, but the point is that there used to be an awareness of what it meant to be well aligned. In the upper classes this awareness was consciously recognised and strived for; in other classes it was perhaps less of a conscious consideration, but still very much a feature of everyday living.

We cannot help but copy those around us. If they stand well, sit well, and move with grace and poise, then so will we. Our elders set the example and we follow. We are easily conditioned creatures until we make a conscious effort to change ourselves.

The 1930s had a depression – but the 20s had their own slump!

Around 1920, a greater influence than the good example of our parents and grandparents hit the scene: the media. The mass production of magazines and newspapers meant that new influences infiltrated our lives on a grand scale. In this case, the expanding influence of the fashion industry and the power of publishing created a new sense of identity for upwardly mobile adults.

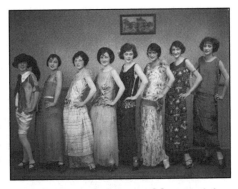

Suddenly, new images were flashed around the world – enticing pictures of 'cool', snazzy, debonair young men and women. They were startling in appearance: they looked different, acted differently, spoke differently, danced differently, and dressed differently; however they also stood differently, sat differently and walked differently. All these things marked them out as 'bright young things' and 'young thrusters'. They became the poster boys and girls of a new generation.

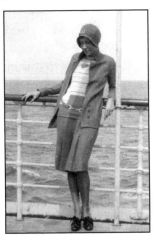

A 'hip' young thing

If you have ever looked at old black and white photographs (pre-1920) you might have been struck by how rigid and stiff characters in portraits and group photos look compared with those we might see today. You might think how uptight, fixed and straight this pre-Great War generation looks to our modern sensibilities. You might take this as evidence of how much more 'relaxed' we are these days. You might also conclude that there is a connection between our more open, less hierarchical society and the stiff, inflexible way this older generation appear to hold themselves. Their lives look more sombre and serious than ours.

Certainly I had all these thoughts for years, but recognize this now as an absolute fallacy. If there is such a thing as odd behaviour, it is our modern manner.

There's no doubt that this 'black and white' generation had to take life seriously, but surely we do too? In terms of the 'unnatural' rigidity we see in the photos, we simply misunderstand how the nature of photograph taking has changed over the years. In fact I would say it is us who are the anomaly; it is us who have become incredibly casual in front of the lens and put ourselves into positions that, though normal to us, are historically and anatomically odd.

Nowadays we take photos casually, at the drop of a hat, often with mobile phones. For the Victorians and Edwardians, having a portrait photo

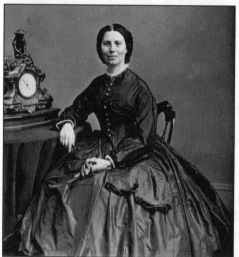

taken was an expensive, lengthy and formal affair. If one was lucky enough to appear in a photo, it was deemed very important to take the opportunity to appear as dignified as possible; dignity demands formality, and formality dictates that one should adopt one's very best pose. Naturally these individuals adopted the poses that they had been taught from an early age were the 'right' ones for persons of 'good standing' (pun intended). A good model was there to follow and, naturally, when the marvel of the camera appeared only the very best pose would do.

Away from the camera they wouldn't have been as strict with themselves, but the baseline positions of good posture that we observe in these photos would have been ever present in their lives.

The fact that these individuals maintained good posture throughout their lives (and didn't just fake it in front of photographers) is evident in the more informal photos we have as records. Photos of bank clerks at work, for example, show that they maintained a proper posture, even though they were required to sit down for up to 12 hours a day. They were capable of doing this without any form of spinal collapse and without the sort of degeneration and pain that is so prevalent today.

This lost generation knew how to sit properly, how to stand properly, how to walk properly – and not even the harmful habit of continual sitting was enough to throw them wildly off-kilter.

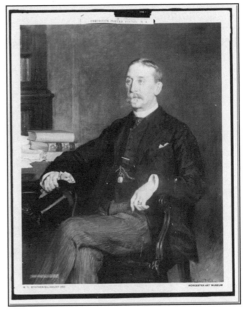

However, the cultural wind change of the 1920s was to change all of that. A brave new generation threw out the old adages, images and examples of their forbearers and set out into the world with a new, daring demeanour: the slouch.

I want to look now at what they actually started to do with their anatomy. In doing so we will start to see what we can do to rectify matters in our own lives. Their problems are our problems, you see. It will become apparent why an intention (or admonition) to 'sit up straight' is really of no help to us.

A very modern stance

You'll come to see that many of the positions we think looked relaxed and comfortable are actually nothing of the sort. They are dominated by a level of tension and discomfort that we have learnt to ignore and accept as normal. Again, we have lost our instincts for what feels right.

Unfortunately, in a book of this sort, it isn't possible to do much more than outline the changes that you could make over a few weeks that would radically transform your relation to gravity. In brief though, there are a series of closely related habits that almost all of us have. These are:

1. *We push our pelvis forward.*

2. *We rock forward so our weight goes over our toes, rather than our heels.*

3. *Our shoulders fall forward, downwards and towards each other (the 'slump') to compensate for our forward-positioned pelvis. (Hump-backed celebrity Quasimodo models this well, but he has many lesser imitators)*

4. *Our head juts forward to compensate for the backward-positioned shoulders.*

The technical name for this is 'kyphosis'. Here is a particularly bad case:

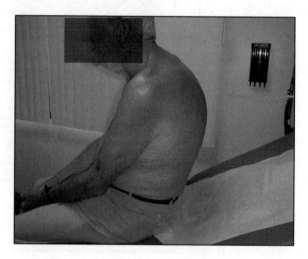

This usually causes the following problems:

1. *The arches of the foot roll in (There is some suggestion that this excessive movement – known as hyper-pronation – could be a congenital issue, but there's plenty of evidence that poor posture and poor shoes are also to blame. We will talk more about shoes later.)*

2. *Knees fall in towards each other when they are bent instead of tracking straight over the toes, as they should ('knock-kneed').*

3. *Lots of muscles and joints stiffen up (too many to list here), especially if you brace your knees to avoid point 2 occurring.*

4. *Some muscles and joints have to become hyper-flexible to compensate for the joints that barely move at all.*

5. *The abdominal area protrudes unattractively, bulging outwards with the weight of its unsupported organs, making the owner look fatter.*

People are often aware that something is amiss – consciously or not – and many do the following to try to negate the issues described above:

1. *They pull their head and shoulders back (to 'stand straight') and their chin IN.*

2. *They puff out their chest and heave their torso up and backwards (to avoid the slouch).*

3. *They suck their stomach in (thinking it makes them look thinner too).*

4. *They lock their knees back to hyper-extend their legs when standing. They brace them outwards when they squat.*

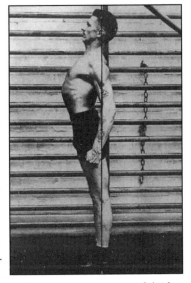

I call the second adaption 'military posture'. If you were ever in the military, you almost certainly do this (unless you ignored your drill sergeant's instructions) but so do lots of people who make a deliberate effort to stand-up straight.

These adaptations can lead to one or more of the following:

1. *A flattened lower back, with a tucked pelvis that's lost the lower curve of its natural 'J' shape. (You must have seen this before with people who appear to have no real bum? Their trousers just hang off the back of their belt.)*

Military stance: many people's idea of how to stand straighter. Notice however, that the hips and chest are much too far in front of the plumb line.

2. *A considerable arch in the mid-back area.*

3. *Lots of additional tension – even more than the amount required to hold the slouch position (hence the false dichotomy between the terms 'ATTENTION' and 'AT EASE' in military parlance. These should be <u>the same thing</u> when an individual is well balanced.)*

People who have pulled themselves up by the bootstraps into what they believe is a better position often look like their posture is better than those who don't; they may even receive regular compliments from ac-

133

quaintances. However, those compliments are just noting the absence of the appearance of the sort of slouch we are used to seeing, and it assumes that what has replaced it is optimal or preferable. In truth, either situation is harmful – however much the 'military posture' might look more pleasing to some eyes.

Here are some pictures of relatively modern but traditional people 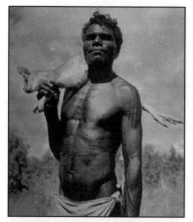 standing or moving well. Their spines maintain a natural 'J' shape. Each body segment is stacked up perfectly over the next, the shoulders are well back and aligned, and their poise radiates grace and confidence.

You'll see from this that most of those who have grown up without western sedentary patterns of movement are much more likely to retain good body alignment – even into old age.

I would surmise that this is for the following reasons:

1. *They have inherited an ancient culture of good posture, which each new generation learns from the last.*

2. *They don't slouch about on chairs.*

3. *They are active for much of the day.*

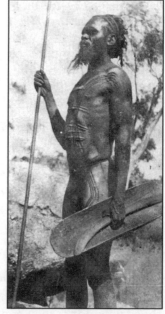

4. *They go barefoot much of the time over varying terrain and retain strength and flexibility in their feet. They certainly don't totter about in high-heels or cushioned trainers, which encourages a horrible displacement of the pelvis.*

5. *They squat regularly and retain flexibility even as they age.*

6. *They don't sleep on excessively soft mattresses, which smother the body's ability to sense where it is in space and*

relax properly. (Mattresses also encourage the body to curl up in a 'C'-shaped, foetal position – a position suitable only for foetuses)

7. *They retain strength across all muscle groupings, not just those isolated at the gym.*

8. *They are rarely obese. (Obesity makes it even harder to fight against gravity once you are at all off-balance).*

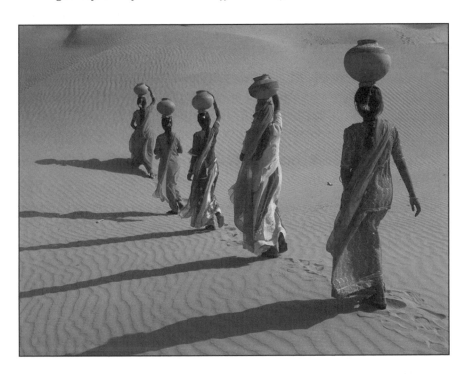

Based on this, I would make the following general suggestions with regard to posture, flexibility and the good movement patterns that stem from this:

1. *Become more aware of your current posture and tension levels. By doing so you will be able to consciously let go of some of the excess effort you are using.*

2. *Learn how to sit well in a chair so you can sit on most chairs for hours without issue when you have to. Learn how to stand well. Learn how to lie in your bed while decompressing your spinal joints and resting fully.*

3. *Squat more often. Before you can squat properly with your heels flat on the ground, you may have to work up to it by squatting with your heels raised on a block.*

4. *Stand or walk around at work when you can. (In California, lots of office workers have begun standing at their workstations rather than sitting)*

5. *Consider a new mattress – not too hard, not too soft. ('Too hard' just means you can't get used to it and sleep eludes you... and you should have gathered by now that you do need your sleep)*

6. *Regain lost flexibility – To help you lose these patterns of excess tension and tightness the years have brought you could consider massage, a specific dynamic stretching routine prescribed just for you by a human movement expert or very knowledgeable personal trainer.*

7. *Learn what good posture looks like, practice to achieve it, and then teach your children.*

8. *Go **barefoot** when you can: on holiday; on the beach; around the house. Buy shoes with plenty of lateral toe space, no heels and a thin sole.*

> Posture might not be 'cool' or in any way 'rock n roll' but to hold what is an evolutionary correct body position does bring numerous benefits to our lives

Go barefoot

Ask anyone and they'll almost certainly agree that going without shoes if one of the best things about being on holiday or on the beach. There's an enormous sense of freedom when we go unshod in the manner in which we came into this world. Even though going barefoot on rough ground can never, on the face of it, be described as more 'comfortable' or 'easy' when compared to wearing the latest hi-tech padded shoes, it does offer a sensory experience much deeper and more 'connected' than a hi-tech training shoe can offer.

We have become prudish and fearful of touching the very earth that supports us.

136

Our feet evolved to be in constant contact with, and receive constant stimuli from, the ground beneath us; a therapeutic massage with every step, if you like. Wearing shoes insulates us from the benefits of this massage and encourages the foot to move in a fixed, inflexible, robotic manner.

In the same way that wearing an injured arm in a sling too long will result in stiff, atrophied muscles and reduced co-ordination, keeping your feet constantly boxed up in 'foot slings' is unnatural and can, over decades, have a seriously detrimental effect on the health of your whole body.

Considering that there are 20 different muscles in the foot, all of which need to work individually and collectively to balance you properly, it's easy to imagine the harm smothering them with a shoe for a lifetime will do. The effects of shoes are seen clearly in feet with collapsed arches, curled toes or bunions – afflictions seldom seen in populations that have never worn shoes.

The knock on effects of all of this can affect the way we stand, move and function. There is excellent evidence for the fact that going barefoot offers the following benefits:

1. *Improved running efficiency*

2. *Improved circulation*

3. *Minimization of back pain*

4. *Enhanced balance and agility*

5. *Stronger calves, feet and foot arches*

The benefits of going barefoot may reach even further. Reflexologists claim to be able to help with both physical and mental ailments by stimulating points on the soles of the feet, and – although to some this may seem a little far-fetched – it does make perfects sense in the light of our body's evolutionary expectations. We have evolved to keep our feet in direct and constant contact with stones, rocks, earth, sand and other types of ground. This friction massages the feet in a variety of different ways. It seems entirely possible that an absence of this sort of stimulation through the wearing of shoes could provoke symptoms that could be helped with intelligent application of skilled, targeted massage.

Proponents of 'Earthing' take this point of view to another level again. They point out that throughout history humans walked barefoot and slept on the ground. They place huge value on the need for humans to spend as much time in contact with the natural earth as possible. Being insulated from the earth by rubber or plastic shoes and man-made surfaces, they believe, breaks the essential healing current of energy that otherwise flows between the earth and our bodies.

The science behind these claims is in its infancy, so instead of waiting for solid proof, why not test it yourself and see how it feels to you? Sling your shoes, get outside and walk on real earth, grass, mud, stones or sand. If it feels great and makes you feel happier, what else matters?

Just watch out for the doggy doo-doos!

The human foot has evolved for more than four million years to do its job without interference from shoes, so why do we continue to wear the latest high-tech shoes that only force us further from the way nature intended?

When you really must wear shoes (even the hardiest bare-footer 'shods up' sometimes), then maybe you could take a look at what has

become known as 'minimalist footwear'; shoes that have only a minimal impact on the way the foot operates. Minimalist footwear is amazingly comfortable and performs brilliantly under any conditions.

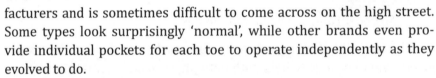

Most minimalist footwear worth its salt comes from small 'niche' manufacturers and is sometimes difficult to come across on the high street. Some types look surprisingly 'normal', while other brands even provide individual pockets for each toe to operate independently as they evolved to do.

Ok, perhaps they're not always the perfect fashion statement for everyone, and they're sure to attract the funny looks worn to a wedding, but they're great outdoors, in a wood, walking through fields, climbing trees, or rocks, or even in the water.

To learn more about these fantastic minimalist shoes and the benefits are of 'barefootness' visit www.instinctive-fitness.com where we compare many of the options available.

We got on to barefooting by considering the importance of great posture. Optimal posture also promotes great flexibility, and together they create a noticeably superior level of structural integrity and strength. Like it or not, 'posture' is undoubtedly the unshakable base upon which all physical movements are built and is a serious weapon in holding back the ravages of old-age. The liveliest pensioners are never those that are hunched over and struggling along; rather they are the ones who still exhibit an erect, upright carriage. At the other end of the scale, most of the best athletes the world has known have had postures that set them apart from the common riff-raff.

So by all means hang your jeans low and adopt a fashionable 'street' slump for a night on the tiles; but, come morning, please re-adopt the stance nature intended.

The next chapter will pull the rug out from under the feet of the fitness industry's answer to everything: that paying for a gym subscription is the one-stop shop for health and wellbeing.

Key chapter points:

- *Relearn good posture to remain mobile for an extra decade or two*
- *Squat more often*
- *Avoid chairs where possible until you can sit properly*
- *Find opportunities to exercise barefooted or in minimalist shoes*
- *Try getting your feet onto real soil.*

CHAPTER EIGHT

The Gym Won't Help (Much)

"Whoso would be a man, must be a non-conformist"
Ralph Waldo Emerson

The florescent lit, pounding music, lycra-donning fiesta that is the local gym is often considered by many people to be the number one resource to improve themselves physically. With thousands of people handing over their credit card details for a subscription each year, a modern gym jammed full of fancy-looking machinery that goes 'beep' and a slick sales team to make grand promises is all too often seen as the easiest route to our modern day quest for fitness.

One of the biggest problems with gyms is that, with all those machines churning away in such a predicable repetitious manner, they're actually just *not that much fun*. So after the initial enthusiasm-filled visits, the shine quickly wears off and the excuses are soon being pulled out of the bag more often than the sweatbands.

The reasons people quit are many, but most boil down to two simple points:

1. *They don't like going.*

2. *They don't achieve the results they want.*

If that sounds like your experience, then the first thing you need to know is that it's not your fault. It is part and parcel of the business model of the gym that you signed up to that you're likely to stop attending soon. It's also expected that, to avoid the stigma of being shown up as a proven 'quitter', you're unlikely to be brave enough to cancel your subscription with any great speed.

Seriously, it's not your fault if you're fat, and it's not your fault if you don't like the gym, don't exercise, don't like your body, or can't get the results you want – and here's why.

141

There's little in a gym that connects with a human being's innate instincts, other than their unfortunate propensity to be attracted towards the empty promise of a quick fix. That's why it's both so hard to get results and so hard to keep going.

I bet it comes as quite a relief to hear that the cards are inordinately stacked against you when it comes to following this attractive, conveniently packaged path to fitness. Ultimately, you should accept that commercial gyms are founded on a business model that doesn't try as hard to help you as it does to separate you from your cash. However, to be fair, the modern gym wasn't actually developed with *you* in mind at all.

In pursuit of... 'muscliness'

Long before 'normal' people went to gyms, machines like the ones you see in every modern gym facility were developed for making muscles all big and puffy – for obtaining that certain macho appearance. People who liked this look and adopted this hobby became known as 'bodybuilders'. They are a very specific type of person with very specific needs: usually men looking for a very particular 'extreme' look. Bodybuilding isn't about health; it isn't about flexibility or stamina, energy or even strength. It's just about *huge* muscles.

Body builders don't want to feel healthier. They don't want to move better. They don't even want to be any stronger. There's nothing in particular they want to be able to do better except to look 'buff' in a tiny pair of shorts on the beach or in the locker rooms.

There is nothing that they won't do in the pursuit of greater muscle mass. They will take dangerous steroids that compromise their health; eat huge quantities of food of dubious quality; and often refrain from any other form of exercise at all lest they burn precious calories they need for muscle growth. They will spend money on fake tan and baby oil, which they will cover themselves with – anything that will get them closer to their ideal muscle-bound image.

To achieve this look, 'special' machines were developed that were capable of isolating each muscle. Over the last 30 years, however, these same machines have been used to commercialise the gym 'experience', convincing a wider public that these facilities fulfill our need for regular movement. Despite throwing the doors open to a wider public, gyms remain a facility designed for the likes of these bodybuilding men, not for meeting the needs of more typical individuals who desire weight loss, strength, balance, flexibility and better health.

So really, it's horses for courses. If you're looking for humungous muscles, get down the gym, get on the 'pec-deck' or Smith machine, and make sure you take whatever sugar-filled, meal-replacement packet they want to sell you too. If however you want to be agile, supple, energetic, stronger, leaner and fitter in a real world way, perhaps you need to look elsewhere.

The blind leading the blind

Go into almost any gym in the country and you'll see the same thing: people dabbling about nervously; people fighting strong feelings of self-consciousness (reinforced by ubiquitous mirrors); and people doubting what they are doing and wondering what on earth they are doing there. As a gym newbie, we suspect everyone else knows what they are doing and is quietly laughing at us.

With a bit more time spent learning the ropes, we inevitably settle in and those feelings subside, often to be replaced with those of boredom. We wrongly thought in the early days that we would grow to like it when we saw results but, sooner rather than later, the realisation dawns that our dream of a miraculous body transformation isn't just around the corner.

Typically we'll have been diligently following the routine set up by a gym instructor. Probably one with only a few weeks' training who, even if he knows better, has little option but to prescribe the exercises he has been told he should include in everyone's programme. He might tell you that his programme is just for you, but actually, like the cog in the machine his is, he churns out the same exercises for every gym member, merely varying the number of reps and sets depending on whether you described yourself as a beginner or an intermediate in your induction.

Most of the exercises he'll get you to do will be one of two types a) largely useless, or b) dangerous.

Most exercises will be of type 'a' – a few are type 'b'. The only exception to the uselessness of the programme is if you are actually a body-builder and are beginning a serious, six-meal-a-day, extreme nutritional programme to try to inflate your muscles to look a bit stronger.

So there they are, blindly following a gym routine founded on repetition, routine, drudgery, ineffectiveness and a little old-fashioned narcissism just because they know no better. What a waste of time and money.

Not understanding what a fruitless, one-sided deal they've signed up to, they trustingly put all their fitness eggs in one gym-shaped basket. But because they hate every second, they quickly stop going. However, they don't cancel their membership because to do so would be to admit defeat; to concede that they will never get fit and that they're a hopeless, miserable failure. Instead they carry on paying for a service that they don't use, with the optimistic delusion that one day they'll return and make it work. From the gym owner's point of view though, this cracking little system works brilliantly.

Statistically about 80% of gym users are absent on any given day from the gym for which they pay an on-going membership.

All this suits the gym owner just fine. In fact, their worst nightmare is their gym becomes popular and everyone starts actually turning up – they haven't possibly got room. Instead, they hope that the *idea* of the gym stays popular; the belief that the gym is the only way to a better quality of wellbeing stays entrenched in our conditioned minds, and they can continue to routinely charge us for this sorry state of affairs.

But beware, if you do go, don't take any cash. Should you have the gall to turn up, they then want to squeeze a bit more out of your pocket by selling you some more stuff that you really don't need: dodgy protein shakes, snack bars, supplements, and the services of 'personal trainers' who'll follow you around watching you do the same exercises you've always done.

Strength is an all-in team effort

The obvious thing that anybody with eyes in their head will quickly notice is that gyms are filled with machines. The machines purport to get you fit, one muscle at a time. Each is designed to isolate individual muscles and exercise them separately from the surrounding ones.

Isn't it ironic that people go to the gym to get mobile again when all the machines are static and fixed to the floor? There's little genuine movement to be seen at all.

Take, for example, the leg extension machine. This is a bench over which your leg hangs. The leg is then extended until it is straight whilst overcoming the inertia posed by the weight resisting this movement. It only really works one muscle: the Rectus Femoris. Yet at the front of your upper leg alone there are six different muscles, and each must work together in unison to be effective in any real-life task or sport. So in fact the exact circumstances that this machine contrives to produce – where one muscle stands alone to do all the work – don't exist anywhere else.

Typically, the result of training on a machine is the targeted muscle becomes filled with additional fluids, making it look bigger and stronger – though increases in actual strength are often minimal. When this happens, you are, for a brief moment, a bodybuilder.

Now this might not sound too bad a compromise for the ease of using a nice machine. But here's the thing. This sort of exercise is totally unnatural. There is nothing else you will ever do in your life where your leg operates in this way. There is never another time out in the real world when you will ever do anything like this again.

Movement in general involves moving or carrying objects or the body along some prescribed, non-linear route. (Think back to the days of hunting and gathering.) To do this we must coordinate *all* the muscles of the body together at the *same* time, balancing ourselves whilst creating the force necessary to make the intended movement and, with practice, showing grace, efficiency and great posture.

In any real life movement our body works as a whole. Almost all of the other muscles contribute to assist balance and support the whole body for every movement we make. Machines, however, isolate muscles and fix our joints in space apart from the one being worked. In doing so, they produce a response which does not improve anything other than the quality of 'puffiness' that the targeted muscle exhibits, and a marginally–elevated ability to perform *just that one exercise*.

Think of muscle isolation exercises like training a regiment of soldiers individually on a distance-learning package, and expecting them to march in time on pass out day.

If you've ever wondered how after a 12-week gym programme you still find it just as hard to lift the shopping out of the boot, here's your answer: you've hardly improved the strength of any whole groups of muscles at all – and there's been no improvement in the synchronisation of the muscle groups involved in this whole body lifting task. Strength is just as much about improved co-ordination as it is about genuine muscle growth. The swollen muscle effect may look very impressive, but is little more than a vanity project.

In this sort of restricted environment no real 'learning' happens, not to mention no real engagement with the environment. Our gym user knows the machine will work exactly as it did last time and that there is no need to be fully present in mind and body in the same way that a hunter-gatherer must fully engage with the task at hand, while simultaneously keeping awareness open for threats at all times.

So, why are gyms filled with machines if they aren't much use to most of us? It's simple really; the reason is that it is the best way to justify the prices they charge. They give you something very obvious to see when you show up and, if you believe that using such machines is the only useful way to exercise, it reinforces the idea that you can't possibly get fit anywhere else. After all, where would you put all the machines that are needed?

Gyms are good for cardio right?

Ah, but what about the **'cardio' machines**, you ask. Surely the stair climber, the cross trainer, and the stationery cycle are good for burning off fat and strengthening my heart and lungs? Well, maybe. It would be mad to suggest you'd be better off at home on the sofa, but there are still some serious reservations about these machines.

Firstly, they're dull. Duller than a dull day in Dulwich! Being stationary, you are faced with an unchanging view for long periods of time. This really isn't very natural. You've probably noticed that when you walk or cycle outdoors normally, the scenery tends to trundle on past you? Not so in the gym. You do sometimes get a mini-television to watch though. This will ensure that there is no way that your mind can be fully involved in the present moment and engaged with the activity you are mindlessly pursuing.

Secondly, you're indoors, yet cardiovascular exercise presents the best opportunity to get outside the concrete cages we surround ourselves with all day long. Getting outdoors, ideally into a natural environment, is one of the most crucial things to do to boost your metabolic rate and raise serotonin and Vitamin D levels. This is hardly an arcane secret: it's not only backed by science but also the good instincts of those city office workers who try to get to the park in their lunch break. They know from experience that their afternoon will be the better for it with higher levels of energy, motivation and drive.

What is less well known is that there is a growing number of people attesting to the existence of "Nature Deficit Disorder" which appears to affect many people from urban areas who don't get a sufficient dose of mud, leaves, trees, insects, wind, temperature change, sunshine and other facets of a real environment – things that our ancestors interacted with every day of their lives.

Others have dismissed the idea that this should be considered a disorder, citing a lack of evidence. All I know is that most of the happy times of my life have been outdoors, and I think that's no coincidence. I am always happier at the end of a walk in the woods than I am when I set off. Never have I returned to the house miserable, wishing I'd covered the same distance at a gym.

Thirdly, most of these machines, apart from the treadmill, are non-weight bearing. Now this can be a good thing if you are injured. However it's well known that an absence of weight-bearing activity leads to a weakening of the bones and connective tissues, and increased incidences of falls and broken bones in later life. So it is just possible that the cross-trainer isn't the wonder machine it is often painted as.

The fourth reason is that the machines are so often used competitively. We compete with ourselves, we compete with the machine and we compete with the person next to us. This isn't useful for cardio. Cardio should be conducted at an easy, conversational pace so that we finish feeling more energised than when we started. However, gyms and the nature of cardio machines encourage us to push, push and push – until we're ready to drop.

Now this isn't something a human being should choose to do regularly. If you're not sure about this, check out the health record of most world-class endurance athletes. Despite being awesomely fit, they are often on the edge of breakdown, their immune systems stretched to the limit to counter the physical and mental stresses to which they subject themselves. Our early ancestors would certainly not have seen the point of this and would have sensibly chosen to save their energy for emergencies or activities with more intrinsic meaning.

Finally, most cardio is unnaturally repetitive. Even on the treadmill – yes, you're running which is good – but every step is exactly like the last. There is no texture to the run. It's a sheer slog. The ground underneath your feet is identical for every step, meaning the tiny muscles in your feet are not encouraged to work hard to adjust to constantly changing terrain. I learnt the subtle but powerful difference this challenging change in terrain made over the weeks in Africa crossing stony, uneven ground.

Beware of your metabolism

Now I'm certainly not against running. I love it. What I see as harmful is the 'chronic' form of cardio (in the form of running, bicycling, or whatever) that most people adopt. If you're out of breath for extended periods of time, you're doing yourself no long-term favours. You can't even expect to burn off more fat this way. You would be shocked at how much time you have to spend exercising to burn off the calories in just a small sandwich, but that's not the only reason that relying on tough, long cardio sessions to lose weight is pure folly.

At higher speeds our metabolism switches from burning fat as its primary fuel, to glucose. This means that glucose (the sugar that gets stored in the muscles) gets depleted, a situation that our body doesn't take kindly to. Its response is to desperately recoup what's been lost and to do its best to prevent this situation happening again. So it increases appetite over the next 24 hours.

The result of all this stock depletion is: **You end up actually eating *more* after this sort of exercise and usually adding *more* weight to your poor, burdened frame.** I have read that the average body fat percentage of runners at running clubs is 22% (a bit chubby). Should we not expect this to be much lower if regular, extended, effortful running was a helpful adjunct to weight loss?

Therefore, as a rule of thumb, when exercise is extensive (25 minutes plus) it should be so dead easy that, should you choose, you could keep it up all day. But when exercise is short and intensive it should be exhilarating, stimulating, fun and BRIEF.

So far I've only detailed what I consider to be wrong with what actually happens at the average gym. What should also be thrown into the mix is what's missing from almost everybody's gym experience:

Missing in action

- *Balance and agility – You'll never see anyone doing anything balance related in the gym, except leaning against the water cooler.*

- *Bodyweight work – being able to handle our own bodyweight well is a prerequisite for living well and performance in sport. You'll rarely see anyone do so much as a pull-up in a gym.*

- *Flexibility and posture – although gym programmes usually toss in a few stretches for good measure, these are usually inappropriate and never lead to long-term improvements in range of movement.*

- *A suitable dietary approach for weight loss, health and better body composition. Most gyms offer no advice, or simply echo the government's failed 'low-fat, healthy grains' approach.*

- *Confidence in challenging, three-dimensional movements, which require concentration and improved coordination to perform. The body needs to be challenged in three different directions (forward and back, side to side, and rotationally) in order to develop as a whole unit.*

- *Support – it's called a 'health and fitness club' but, let's face it, there's nothing 'club-like' about it at all. It'll take months to get to know anyone and when they do speak to you it'll probably just be to check that you're finding it as fruitless a process as they are.*

We'll finish this chapter by acknowledging that there are a few gyms out there that are not guilty of much of the above. They are few and far between, but if you can get to a **Crossfit** style gym you'll do pretty well for yourself. They have few machines (although they are strangely fond of rowing) and rely on natural, three-dimensional movements that emphasise strength, power, balance, endurance and agility. Their workouts are very tough and rugged however. You can easily find yourself overtraining in a place like this. It's also important that you take care to use good form on every exercise or you may find yourself quickly injured (like too many overly-competitive adherents). On the plus side, many have a good grasp of decent nutrition, and most Crossfit gyms actually want you to turn up as their business model isn't as cynical as the mainstream ones. So yes, there *are* some pitfalls to beware – but it's all good, natural movement so your efforts won't be as wasted as they are in a conventional gym.

So Crossfit gyms get the IF stamp of approval, but otherwise give the gym a miss. If you love it, it *is* possible to use one sensibly, but most of the good stuff you could do at home, in the garden or in a park.

Key chapter points:

- *Regular gyms are not designed for you, but for bodybuilders with very specific, extreme aesthetic goals (which only work with extreme nutritional plans).*

- *Gyms primarily want your money, not your attendance. (It's in their business model that most of their customers won't attend.)*

- *Most gym equipment is hopeless for achieving the goals of ordinary people.*

- *Machines isolate muscle function, meaning there's very little transferral of ability to your own life. The best you might get is 'good at gym'.*

- *Cardio machines are a wasted opportunity to get outside and enjoy all the benefits that this brings. They are almost always used incorrectly, so that weight loss is harder and fitness gains are compromised. Overtraining is easy.*

- *Many of your basic fitness needs (three-dimensional balance, agility, power, co-ordination and real-world strength) will not be addressed by a conventional gym or the off-the-peg programme you'll be given.*

- *You're not alone if you dislike the atmosphere in your gym. It's a lonely, soulless place that doesn't fulfill your basic need for real movement.*

CHAPTER NINE

Don't Let Your Government, Doctor, Family or Friends Tell You How to Eat

So you can now see how the natural physical movement and exercise that nature intended us to enjoy has been hijacked and twisted to fill the pockets of a goliath health and fitness industry. But at least the accepted advice on healthy food and nutrition is rock solid, right?

Here we go again...

Actually, no – the muddle we've got ourselves in gets even worse. The advice we're given on good nutrition is also fundamentally flawed, and this chapter is going to expose how society has been sold another big, fat lemon.

The journey of correcting the accepted but flawed conventional wisdom and showcasing *genuinely* healthy food we're about to embark on is going to be another monumental swim against the tide of popular opinion. But please bear with me because, arguably, the food we eat is even *more* important to our looks, weight, mood and overall health than exercise.

Big brother is watching you...eat!

The establishment has spent millions of pounds telling us how we should eat healthily in order to enjoy good health, pumping out fact after fact in the vain hope of reducing the strain on a National Health Service buckling under the weight of citizens who live so long, but are unwell for much of it.

For the last 30 years or so, the British Government and its Department of Health – neither of which seemingly trust you to think for yourself – have generally been singing the same sort of tune, while quietly changing some very important lyrics. We have been told repeatedly, for

151

example, that in order to control our weight and minimise the chance of cardiovascular disease we should eat a **"low-fat, starch-based diet"** and enjoy **"healthy whole grains and vegetables"**.

While this message hasn't really changed for some time, we have been increasingly warned off certain foods like butter, lard, red meat and full-fat milk – and even, at one time, eggs[1] The establishment is still firmly of the position that the saturated fat found in these products are damaging to health.

On the back of these largely unsubstantiated claims – claims which the British public have swallowed whole – other products have appeared to replace these allegedly dangerous products. Examples of these are margarine (which has been around since the last world war but has grown massively in popularity over recent decades), skimmed and homogenised milk, highly processed vegetable oils, artificial sweeteners and a huge number of processed foods and meals.

In general, the British people have taken this anti-fat message to heart and have bought anything in sight with the words 'low-fat' printed on them. In fact we now eat less fat than we have ever done, and we take in most of our calories in the form of starchy breads, pastas, biscuits, pastries, rice and potatoes. The majority of these products are made from grain (potatoes being the exception), and particularly wheat. What all of these products have in common is that they are massively **high-carbohydrate products.**

Carbohydrates are the foods that the body burns by converting it into glucose, which is just another form of sugar, and it then converts that into glycogen, which is stored in the liver and muscles ready to be deployed as energy.

The sugar paradox

The other part of the low-fat message endorsed by our government and health gurus is that we also need to avoid sugar if we hope to improve our health and lose weight. Products like fizzy drinks, ice cream and sweets are widely criticised for the high levels of sugar they contain (and rightly so).

But have you ever noticed the glaring contradiction in this line of thinking though? It should be quite easy to spot from looking at the last few paragraphs. If we get most of our calories from carbohydrates instead of fat, and carbs break down into sugar, then we're going to be inadvertently eating an awful lot of sugar whether we intend to or not. This is the very same sort of sugar that we are told, in the next piece of the confusing puzzle, we should be avoiding.

Now the above is of course a simplified description of the very complicated chemical reactions that go on in the body. I don't want to give the impression that there's nothing more to it than this, but nor do I want to try clumsily offering a first year course in Biochemistry.

However, in essence, the case goes like this: in order to avoid the fat which we are told is bad for us, we are told to eat plenty of carbohydrates. Carbohydrates quickly turn into sugar, a substance we are told by the exact same sources is bad for us. Sugar, if not burned through exercise, encourages the body to store fat. It also disrupts our blood-sugar levels and, in the longer term, moves us steadily in the direction of diabetes. *'Go figure'*, as the Americans are so fond of saying.

You might wonder if this apparent 'Catch 22' is unavoidable though. Perhaps there is no alternative but to turn to this carb-heavy diet if fat is so bad for us; but that's a big 'if', so we'd better examine the evidence for this claim against fat.

Baffled and bamboozled by science?

Today's near-total hysteria about saturated fat and cholesterol all dates from the publication of the (supposedly) scientific paper 'The Seven Countries Study". Published in 1970 by the American doctor **Ancel Keys**. Keys was a great believer that it was fatty cholesterol deposits in the veins and arteries that caused heart disease. He wanted to verify his theory, and so set off to gather the evidence that would prove him right.

It was this 'study' that provided a whole generation of doctors and scientists with supposedly cast-iron facts to beat us with and, in effect, change the nature of the food we would be advised to eat for the next five decades.

In the study, 12,770 men (no women) aged between 40-59 years, were enrolled in seven countries, in four regions of the world (United States, Northern Europe, Southern Europe, Japan). He actually already had the data available for 22 countries from other studies he had completed earlier but for some reason chose to focus just on these seven countries. Because of this, he has been accused, fairly or not, of 'cherry-picking' his data to fit the conclusions he was hoping to be able to make.

His methods of data collection have been relentlessly criticized by plenty of people who know what good studies *should* look like,[2] but nevertheless, he somehow made the link between the consumption of saturated fat and heart disease. His work became the gold standard that informed western dietary opinion for decades.

Even if we suppose that his data collection was sound, there's one very important point to be made here:

Correlation isn't causation

Far too often in science, correlation is mistaken for causation. For example:

Seagulls are often found following fishing trawlers around, so we can tell that trawlers cause the production of seagulls.

(...or perhaps it's the seagulls causing fishing trawlers?)

Both are ridiculous of course; we can understand this on a common sense level; all these factors just occur together because of a third, un-considered variable – in this case, of course, their common presence is explained by a mutual interest in fish. However, we don't generally have the knowledge to spot the same error in specialist areas when dressed up as 'indisputable facts' by supposed experts.

If the scientific community was to really sit up, take notice and take on board the study findings on face value, as researchers Yerushalmy and Hilleboe have pointed out, they should be advising us to eat far *more* total fat. When Keys' data is properly analysed, it shows that, on aver-age, deaths from *all diseases* (not just heart disease) were actually *lower* for those who ate more total fat, animal fat, and animal protein. This meant that statistically, if you want to live longer, and you take Keys' study to heart (pun intended), you need to eat *more* fat.

A critical eye

What throws a dark cloud across the 'Seven Countries Study' is the fact that amongst the evidence in the 22 countries Keys earlier studied was clear findings that actually showed the direct *opposite* to the link the Sev-en Countries Study claimed to find. Amongst the groups excluded from the second study were quite a number that were shown to eat massive quantities of saturated fat and suffered from almost no cardio-vascular disease whatsoever. The omitted data included the diets of the Masai[3] (with a diet dominated by red meat, milk and blood), the Inuit who we've already discussed (who just eat high-blubber animals) and the Tokelau (who get more than 50% of their calories from saturated fat).

It certainly can't be denied that saturated fats are sometimes found in the diet of those people with cardiovascular difficulties, but it doesn't automatically follow that saturated fats *cause* heart disease.

Even now, more than 50 years on from that first fateful paper, few scientists are prepared to stick their head above the parapet and risk the wrath of cozy, accepted opinion. Copycat, sycophantic studies are still being churned out today, scare-mongering about the consumption of red meat. However they consistently fail to account properly for differences between processed meat and healthy, natural meat, and between intensive industrial farming (with its reliance on antibiotics and steroids) and meat provided by properly fed, pastured animals.

These studies also invariably fail to adjust for the fact that the people eating the most meat and fat are usually those also eating the most canned, cured and 'reclaimed' meat, the most junk food, the most hydrogenated vegetable oil, the most salt and sugar, and the most 'messed about with' processed food in general.

The fact is that these studies just aren't good enough. They simply don't factor in all the different variables and, even if they did/could, all they can find is a *link* and, as we showed earlier, a link in no way indicates a *cause*.

Still, as a result of unscientific and insecure studies like these, the British people are now told to eat no more than two portions of red meat a week, avoid butter, and to choose skimmed milk, margarine and vegetable oils instead. In fact we are told to return to a diet pretty similar to the one enforced upon the entire British population during and after the Second World War when sausages, eggs, cheese, butter, bacon and milk were heavily rationed (while fish and fruit were eaten in abundance.) Over a 14 year period this extraordinary experiment involving 50 million people actually coincided with a doubling of cardiovascular disease...but maybe that was just a coincidence?

When the press use phrases like 'artery-clogging, saturated fat', it's easy to see how a natural substance – our body's primary fuel source and a substance from which much of our body is composed – has become so demonised.

This is the point someone normally says, "but saturated fat causes *cholesterol* deposits in the arteries, and excessively high cholesterol can cause heart attacks."

Now here's the strange thing: Keys, the father of sat-fat fears, seemingly didn't have a bad word to say about eating cholesterol. He thought *dietary* cholesterol was pretty much irrelevant. In his paper "The relationship of the diet to the development of atherosclerosis in man," Keys is pretty clear about his views:

*The evidence—both from experiments and from field surveys—indicates that the cholesterol content, per se, of all **natural** diets has no significant effect on either the serum cholesterol level or the development of atherosclerosis in man.*

This topic could expand indefinitely and, if you're still interested, I would point you in the direction of Dr. Malcolm Kendrick's excellent and highly readable book, *The Great Cholesterol Con*.

We'll talk more about cholesterol later, but it's probably fair to say that the production of cholesterol is perhaps the most maligned natural process our body performs. Here again, the latest research suggests that cause and effect have been mixed up. Excess cholesterol does not cause harm to the body at all[4], but is in actual fact the body's attempt to *heal* itself. Instead, it is now becoming increasingly clear that the body produces cholesterol in a controlled and intelligent way to patch up the damage caused to the body by inflammation and oxidation.

Thinking cholesterol causes damage to the body is like believing sticky plasters cause cuts because they are often found together in the same place.

Does it not seem bizarre that red meat with its 'dangerous' cholesterol and 'artery-clogging' fat (the main food source that sustained and nourished us for the vast majority of our evolutionary history) has suddenly, over the last century, become a danger to our health? If this is true, the question is: How did human beings ever survived as a species at all? What's next? Will we decide grass is bad for cows and that primates should avoid fruit?

If the results of all the subsequent studies are viewed not through the lens of one originally flawed theory, but through the open eyes of objectivity, there is plenty of evidence that demonstrates the *benefits* of increased fat and cholesterol in our diets. Again these are just correlations and not proof of cause and effect, but perhaps considering the following will shed some more light:

Naughty, fat munching countries

Between 1958 and 1999, the Japanese doubled their protein intake, ate 400 per cent more fat and their cholesterol levels went up by 20 per cent. If Keys was right, they should have dropped like flies – but did they? No. Their stroke rate, which had been the highest in the world, was reduced sevenfold, while deaths from heart attacks dropped by 50 per cent.

Then there's the French. They eat much more saturated fat than we do in Britain; they smoke more, take less exercise, and have the same cholesterol levels; they also have the same average blood pressure. However, they have considerably lower rates of obesity and one quarter of the rate of heart disease that we do. This fact has confused (and is more often ignored by) so many scientists that it's become known as the French Paradox.

Numerous surveys of traditional populations have yielded statistics that confound all those who have sought to indoctrinate us in the dangers of saturated fat. For example, a study comparing Jews living in Yemen, whose diets contained fats only of an animal origin, to Yemenite Jews living in Israel, whose diets contained margarine and vegetable oils, showed little heart disease or diabetes in the former group but high levels of both diseases in the latter.[5]

A comparison of populations in northern and southern **India** revealed a similar pattern. People in northern India consume 17 times more animal fat but have an incidence of coronary heart disease seven times lower than the people of southern India who lean more towards a vegetarian diet.[6]

The **Masai** and kindred tribes of Africa subsist largely on beef, blood and milk (they drink the blood of their cattle). However they are largely free from coronary heart disease and have excellent blood cholesterol levels.[7]

The **Inuit** eat inordinately large quantities of animal fats from fish and sea animals. Those who still eat the traditional diet are free of disease and exceptionally hardy.[8]

This isn't a case of 'the exception proves the rule'; there are many, many more examples of countries confounding the prejudices of the low-fat propaganda wagon. There's more in the notes at the end of the chapter.[9] And anyway...

How can ancient foods cause a modern disease? Does that really make any sense?

Actually, posed more accurately, the question is: **How can ancient foods that we eat in lower quantities than ever before, be causing modern diseases that we almost never had in the past?**

You only have to look back to the 1930s to find a time when people were eating large amounts of saturated fat in the UK. Even though 'healthy' margarine made from seed-oils hadn't been introduced as a replacement for 'dangerous' butter and lard, there were almost no cases of heart disease or lung cancer, despite the fact that 80% of the population smoked.

However, on the back of Keys' highly dubious study, a whole new approach to dieting was formed and food companies rushed to produce new foods to fulfill the demand for 'healthy', 'low-fat' products and to fill their own coffers. We will look at these some more in Chapter Eight when we consider 'Real Food'.

The sad fact is that there was a need for a study showing fat equals heart attack and, although the results of Keys' study didn't really show that at all, it was enough for the author to appear on the front page of *Time Magazine* and a whole new, low-fat approach to health to be born. The theory that saturated fat is unhealthy was hammered into our consciousness by foul play:

And the 'Lipid Hypothesis' was promoted to 'Lipid Fact'... Magic!

Since that time, led by the USA and the UK, a fifty-year experiment into the effects of this baseless leap into the dark has been running. The findings aren't pretty, as we found in Chapter Three, but too many people in power have a vested interest in the status quo to change tack now.

Is this conspiracy or just plain incompetence?

There's enough here for another book but the usual human failings raise their heads.

Corporate greed – We have devolved responsibility for the quality preparation of our foodstuffs to giant corporations: the supermarkets, the processed food companies and the junk food restaurants. These megalithic monsters have just one intrinsic duty – to deliver their shareholders a juicy bottom line profit, not improved public health or nutrition.

Any profitable company's sole *raison d'être* is to do just that: generate profit. So wherever there are opportunities to cut corners and produce a food product that only looks like a healthy one (but isn't) for less overheads, they will almost always take it. Ker-Ching.

Ignorance – These days cooking and **culinary skills** are rarely passed on with the loving care from one generation to the next as they used to be. People just don't know any better. Who's got time to read books, let alone invest some time and thought into how and what they cook? (Apart from you, dear reader – you brilliant, brainy exception to the rule!)

Gullibility – We tend to be a trusting lot. We glibly assume our government and 'big business' wouldn't do anything *too* awful to us. We tend to actually believe the convenient, cherry-picked science our government passes our direction, and that large, recognised and respected organisations won't lack vital knowledge in matters they are *supposed* to be experts in.

To be fair though, our elected governments and MPs are ordinary people too. Most don't know any better and it is part and parcel of their job to stay onside with 'big industry' and the pressure groups that support them. They won't dare rock the boat or bite the hand that feeds them for fear of a ballot box backlash come the next elections.

Too many influential people and groups have a vested interest in maintaining the status quo. If they *did* happen to stumble across the holy grail of good health – what's the betting they'd shove it straight back into its dusty box and bury it somewhere it could never be found?

The establishment simply has too much invested in the existing state of affairs. Simple, cheap solutions to big problems don't make money for important people and are never going to be welcomed by the people in power.

Sloth – Actually, this isn't a reason at all – so it shouldn't really be on the list. Most people are neither lazy nor slothful – they just lack perspective, knowledge and motivation. Of course people don't *want* to spend their time preparing food at home when they believe that something almost as nutritious and perhaps as tasty can be found in a supermarket ready-made meal. It's not even true to say we don't have enough time in our day; people have just as much time as they've always. In a convenient exception to the world's other terrible inequalities, we all get exactly the same 24 hours each day, whether millionaire or beggar.

The problem is those people who believe they have 'no time to cook' just don't prioritise it highly enough over all the other uses of their time to make it happen. They would rather work longer hours, spend more time socialising, sit in front of the TV, or whatever else. This is of course their choice, but would they make the same choices if they knew the full facts?

Government gaff

It's not the case that our government doesn't care at all for our welfare – because it clearly does – unfortunately. If it *didn't* care, it would keep its dubious health advice to itself and we would all be much better off. No, the problem is that it *does* care for our health (at least a bit) but has two hugely incompatible agendas.

1. *Improving the nation's health*

2. *Raising big companies' profits to strengthen the economy.*

Unfortunately, these objectives are almost totally at odds with one another (or at least they are while all the big money remains in processed foods). Governments are trapped between a big rock and seriously hard place, and someone's definitely not going to be happy.

So rather than make some waves and agree on what's most important, what we've ended up with is some horrible attempt at a compromise: a supposedly 'healthy diet' for the individual which still maximises the profit of big corporations. Hell, even McDonald's and Coca-Cola were allowed to sponsor the London Olympics – an occasion that should celebrate health and vitality, not promote its biggest opponents.

Cronyism and mutual back scratching have run amok in the world of consumer health. The British Nutrition Foundation is the organisation that advises government, schools, industry, health professionals and the public on all matters to do with health and food. It exists, apparently, to deliver "authoritative, evidence-based information on food and nutrition" and claims to be "world class in the interpretation and translation of complex nutritional science."

However, lurking within the 39 members that contribute to the BNF's funding are some multi-billion pound 'food' companies including: Cadbury, Coca Cola, Kellogg's, Northern Foods, Nestlé, McDonald's, PizzaExpress, and most of the main supermarket chains. The former chairman of its board of trustees, Paul Hebblethwaite, was at the very same time wearing another hat: that of Chairman of the Biscuit, Cake, Chocolate and Confectionery Trade Association. Now there's a man who wrestled with a serious conflict of interests!

When this is the sort of 'independent' and 'impartial' advice that drives government policy, are you sure you want to take every last word of it on face value?

This conflict of interest is made even worse by the pharmaceutical companies' obvious vested interest in seeing our poor health continued. In this way they can happily rake in the profits from alleviating our symptoms, while causes remain unaddressed. (The multi-billion pound prescriptions for statins to combat high cholesterol are a prime example of this – even when diet and exercise remain the simple, free and profitless solution to this threat).

In short, we've got ourselves in a right merry mess.

Successive governments have collaborated out of sheer desperation with pressure groups, the medical industry and the self-interest of the processed food industry. In doing so, they have effectively told us what to think and closed our minds to considering other possibilities, even when it is only too apparent to those who dare look that this mass-engineered experiment has not worked. The end result is that the whole way we think about health and weight loss has become tainted.

The definition of insanity widely attributed to Einstein's was *"continuing to do the same thing but expecting a different result"*. Perhaps we should be reminded of this while countries like the UK continue to follow their government's advice to cut healthy fats from their diets, hoping that suddenly, as if by magic, we're all going to get slimmer and healthier.

The truth finally wakes from its slumber

There have, of course, been other opinions expressed over the years that have been systematically shouted down to save face and maintain the status quo. However, these voices are now becoming increasingly more numerous, and are at last starting to be heard.

The largest of these is the **low-carb movement**, which has grown over the last 10 years to become the biggest thorn in the side of 'conventional wisdom'. This new movement has gathered followers through the medium of the Internet and huge quantities of positive anecdotal testimonials. More recently, meta-studies (studies of studies) of diets have also shown 'low-carb diets' to be more successful than 'low-fat' as a weight loss approach.[10]

At last, it seems that, although the establishment is not yet ready to listen, we as a population are crying out to try something different. And this means, for the moment, ignoring the official line that stubbornly refuses to change – despite being ridiculed daily by the ever-growing statistics that prove its abject failure.

Key chapter points:

- *Listen to advice, but decide for yourself on matters of importance. Logic is better than blind faith, but self-experimentation can be the ultimate litmus test.*

- *Bad science and a desperate establishment have brainwashed us into fearing fat. Fat is your friend. You're made of the stuff – it's supposed to be your principal fuel.*

- *The 'low-fat and healthy grains' ideology has failed us. Look around you.*

- *You can't trust the food industry to feed you well. They care about their profit, not your health.*

- *You can't trust the government either; it's in the thrall of the big food giants and their manipulative lobby groups.*

- *Low-carb is the future, but don't wait to be told 'officially'. The establishment hates U-turns.*

- *All diets, apart from the one endorsed by 2.5 million years of evolution, are based on fads not facts.*

References:

1. Recently however, the government health warning on eggs has been rescinded (read: 'U-turn'). Fears about eggs raising cholesterol levels were acknowledged to be erroneous now that it has been accepted that eggs are only high in one particular sort of cholesterol, one that they now concede isn't harmful. The other, they're still not happy about.

2. Wikipedia (2012) Uffe Ravnskov [Online] Available at: http://en.wikipedia.org/wiki/Uffe_Ravnskov#Investigation_of_the_Lipid_Hypothesis.2C_or_.22Diet-Heart.22_Idea

3. Ho K-J et al. (1971) "Studies on the Masai." Archeological Pathology, 91:387; Mann GV,

et al. (1972) "Atherosclerosis in the Maasai." American Journal of Epidemiology, 95:26-37

4. The Great Cholesterol Con by Dr. Malcolm Kendrick (7 Jul 2008); and also, Pinckney ER, Pinckney C (1973) The Cholesterol Controversy, Sherbourne Press, Los Angeles

5. Cohen A (1963) "Fats and carbohydrates as factors in atherosclerosis and diabetes in Yemenite Jews." Am Heart J, 65:291

6. Malhotra, S, (1968) Indian Journal of Industrial Medicine, 14:219

7. Ho K-J et al. (1971) "Studies on the Masai." Archeological Pathology, 91:387; Mann GV, et al. (1972) "Atherosclerosis in the Maasai." American Journal of Epidemiology, 95:26-37

8. Price, W (1945) DDS, Nutrition and Physical Degeneration, Price-Pottenger Nutrition Foundation, San Diego, CA, 59-72.

9. Several Mediterranean societies have low rates of heart disease even though fat — including highly saturated fat from lamb, sausage and goat cheese—comprises up to 70% of their caloric intake. The inhabitants of Crete, for example, are remarkable for their good health and longevity. Willett WC et al. (1995) "Mediterranean diet pyramid: a cultural model for healthy eating" Am J Clin Nutr, June 1995, 61:1402S – 1406S; Perez-Llamas F et al (1996) "Estimates of food intake and dietary habits in a random sample of adolescents in south-east Spain" J Hum Nutr Diet, Dec 1996, 9:6:463-471; Alberti-Fidanza, A, et al, Eur J Clin Nutr, Feb 1994, 48:2:85-91
A study of Puerto Ricans revealed that, although they consume large amounts of animal fat, they have a very low incidence of colon and breast cancer. Fernandez NA (1975) "Nutrition in Puerto Rico" Cancer Res, 35:3272- 3291; Martines I et al. (1975) "Cancer Incidence in the United States and Puerto Rico" Cancer Res, 35:3265 -3271.
A study of the long-lived inhabitants of Soviet Georgia revealed that those who eat the most fatty meat live the longest. Pitskhelauri GZ (1982) The Long Living of Soviet Georgia, Human Sciences Press, New York, NY.
In Okinawa, where the average life span for women is 84 years—longer than in Japan—the inhabitants eat generous amounts of pork and seafood and do all their cooking in lard. The Swiss live almost as long on one of the fattiest diets in the world. Tied for third in the longevity stakes are Austria and Greece—both with high-fat diets. Moore TJ (1990) Lifespan: What Really Affects Human Longevity, Simon and Schuster, New York, NY.
None of these studies is mentioned by those urging restriction of saturated fats. Other than Keys, the 'Framingham Study' is always cited as the 'evidence' for the flawed Lipid Hypothesis. However, after 40 years, the director stated: "The more saturated fat one ate, the more cholesterol one ate, the more calories one ate, the lower the person's serum cholesterol...we found that the people who ate the most cholesterol, ate the most saturated fat, ate the most calories, weighed the least and were the most physically active."

10. Hession M et al. (2008) "Systematic review of randomized controlled trials of low-carbohydrate vs. low-fat/low- calorie diets in the management of obesity and its comorbidities". Obesity Reviews 10(1): 36-50.

CHAPTER TEN

Natural Food

"Let food be thy medicine and medicine be thy food"
Hippocrates
(The Father of Modern Medicine)

"Just Eat Naturally Edible Food"

That's it. If you've taken on board everything you learned in the previous chapter, that's all I should need to write, and this chapter could be really short. But perhaps we should expand somewhat for those who still consider a box of cereal a 'healthy' option.

To put it simply: if your ancient hunter-gatherer ancestors didn't eat it – and you want to have the same magnificent health and longevity that they did – you should probably refrain as well. So the ever-so-slightly expanded version of my advice is:

DON'T EAT grains, sugar, margarines, vegetable oils, and other industrially processed foods.

There, it's said, point made; now you're ready to follow this great advice and discover that everything that you might hope for from a good eating plan is yours: low body-fat, good health, energy, optimal mood – everything.

What? You're not buying that? You say that your daily loaf is full of whole grains and your box of Frosted Flakes is fortified with iron and minerals so they must be good, right?

Here, put simply, is the situation and the problem:

The most attractive tasting food in our natural environment was good for us. The most attractive tasting food in a modern day environment very probably isn't.

As human beings, we evolved to eat anything around us that didn't present insurmountable toxic defences. In terms of foods this meant that we could eat animals (including seafood), most non-toxic insects, and non-toxic plants, seeds, nuts and roots.

Humans (in the form of homo sapiens) have been on the planet for the last 200,000 years. And for 190,000 of these we were big game hunters and foragers who consumed meat and plants in roughly equal measure.

Raw food uses up a lot of calories just in its digestion. Once the use of fire for cooking was discovered it became easier for us to consume more calories, because heating helps speed up the digestion of meats and plants.

We were sub-consciously driven to hunt, kill or forage the most nutritious and calorie dense fare because, quite simply, they were the things that tasted and smelled best to us. Our senses were our most incredibly accurate and potent guide to what to eat and we trusted them implicitly. *Evolution ensured that what tasted good to us, really _was_ good for us.* We could even say there was a simple, dependable equation that governed our subconscious instinct to survive:

Taste Good = Is Good.

This 100% natural, freshly killed prey, or straight-out-of-the-soil vegetation or foraged honey, insects, fruit or berries, were the only foods we lived on for 190,000 years, right up until the agricultural revolution. At this point – going back only 5% of our time on the planet as fully formed humans and 0.4% of our time as hominids – some bright spark discovered a way of making foods previously inedible to us just about partially edible. This changed everything.

The simple and reliable equation above now became somewhat twisted and less clear-cut:

Taste Good = Sometimes Good, Sometimes Bad – Who knows?

It was the discovery of grain processing that signaled the start of a breakdown in our ability to unthinkingly trust our instincts and our own senses. Suddenly something that tasted and smelled good sometimes *wasn't* actually all that good for us at all. With limited nutritional value and a remnant of their toxic defences still intact, these grains began to fool our taste buds and replace many of the foods that we *should* have been hardwired to seek out.

166

In a nutshell, before agriculture and processed foods, anything that we could find about us in the natural environment that looked appealing, smelt attractive and tasted good, *was* good; after the advent of agriculture this was no longer necessarily true.

This compromise in our ability to trust our inherent taste for what's good for us still lives with us today. Our inbuilt, 'gut instinct' to seek out the tastiest things often leads us woefully astray from the foods that evolution dictates we should thrive on. In a modern supermarket there are thousands of artificial products that will provide hyper-stimulation to our palate and ensnare us in a vicious cycle of addictive consumption. In the distant past, only seasonal honey or rare tree saps with an incredibly sweet taste might have been capable of producing this sort of knee-jerk desire – a desire that the modern consumer has to learn to temper with self-discipline and common sense.

> *"No, darling – three packets of Haribo is quite enough for your breakfast..."*

It's also the unfortunate case that the consumption of these sugary and 'carby' temptations provides a stimulus to the body that overrides another important instinct: our innate sense of when we've had enough to eat. This is completely overridden by the sensory hit that these larger-than-life foodstuffs produce in our mouths. The natural feeling of fullness only occurs much later in the eating process, once we have eaten a whole lot more than we otherwise would have done.

Appetite dysregulation and a desensitized palate are two of the biggest challenges for anyone looking to lose weight and get healthy. For many people, ordinary, unprocessed foods have lost their lustre and they no longer know when they've had enough to eat.

Even a whole grain isn't a healthy grain

It is an undisputed fact that grains (along with beans) could simply not be consumed by human beings until the advent of organised agriculture. As already discussed, fossil records clearly show human health and longevity plummeted when we stopped consuming the edible flora and fauna found around us, and started farming crops instead. We can tell from their bones that agriculturalists were shorter, had more cavities, smaller brains, and had weaker skeletons than hunter-gatherers. Life expectancy also dropped dramatically.

Marta Lahr, co-director of Cambridge University's "Leverhulme Centre for Human Evolutionary Studies," states that "when modern humans, Homo sapiens, first appeared around 200,000 years ago they were tall and muscular...The fossil evidence for the next 190,000 years is patchy, but shows that humans remained tall and robust until about 10,000 years ago when many populations show reduced stature and brain size. It is a striking change..."

Fast forward 200,000 years to the early 20th century when our diet took another turn for the worse. At this point food production became fully industrialised, leading to the appearance of vegetable oil, fluffy white flour (originally produced specifically to prevent factory workers taking expensive toilet breaks), and inexpensive, refined sugar products. As industrialisation grew, it concocted a host of new products, which we naively allowed to be called 'foods'. (It shouldn't come as news to you that, for example, jelly is not a real food, even though all of its constituent parts can be found in nature. It is a manufactured food – a product of food, certainly – but not a food in itself.)

The true scope and limits of the human diet for better or worse was mapped out in the 1930s by an extraordinary gentleman called **Dr. Weston Price**. Known as the 'Charles Darwin of Nutrition," Price was a scientific explorer in every sense of the phrase; a true maverick prepared to think outside of the rules of his time. The good doctor dedicated a *decade of his life* to travelling the world scrutinizing and recording the diets of societies that had been kept totally isolated from the outside modern world. He recorded all his findings meticulously and presented them to the wider public in book: *Nutrition and Physical Degeneration*. (You can still order this book on Amazon today. It still sells well.)

Over the course of his long investigations, he sought out and studied fourteen entirely self-contained, untouched communities – from Irish to Eskimos to Africans – and perhaps surprisingly noted that in almost every case all members of the tribe or village enjoyed robust health into their 80s and often well beyond. Price discovered them to be almost entirely free of chronic disease, dental decay and mental illness. He found they lived fully active, healthy lives right up until the end of their days.

When he compared these people to those inhabitants of the same country who had abandoned their traditional ways of eating (and indeed living), he found a glaring chasm. These people enjoyed none of the health benefits that were so clearly identified in their non-industrialised counterparts who maintained their ancient culinary traditions. Their reliance on the new foods of the industrialised revolution – refined grains, canned foods, pasteurized milk and sugar – meant that they led lives seriously compromised in health and vitality and invariably died decades earlier. Consistently, he also discovered the presence of rampant infectious disease, degenerative illness, infertility and facial and dental deformity.

One of Price's most astonishing discoveries was the difference between Australian Aborigines who maintained their ancestral diet and those who changed to the new diet of the white, western colonialists. The second group, living on sugar, white flour and canned goods, developed rampant tooth decay and diseases of every type pretty quickly, while the former group, on their traditional diet, continued to enjoy uninterrupted health and vitality.

For more information check out the Western Price Foundation http://www.westonaprice.org/

Certainly, grains such as wheat, corn, barley and rye have allowed us to feed millions more people on our ever-populated planet through the management of their growth. The issue is this: if what Dr. Price and an increasing number of modern scientists are now saying is correct, most of these neological (new) foods are still partially toxic to human beings. There are now plenty of studies that show that it is these foodstuffs that are causing untold damage to our gut lining, to our immune systems, to our waistlines and to our health.[1]

Now if this is really the case, then this represents (as Al Gore might say) a seriously 'inconvenient truth'. However, there are a burgeoning number of nutritionists, researchers, scientists, and doctors who are, with heavy hearts, coming around to this uncomfortable point of view. The Paleo Diet, upon which the Instinctive Fitness approach leans heavily, eschews modern foods in favour of Paleolithic ones, and is one of the fastest growing dietary trends in the world. In the USA, it has gained a sizeable following as people abandon the failed advice of their government in favour of eating patterns that have been the foundation of every human being's development since before written history.

If this is true, why haven't we all heard about it before?

Perhaps it's because cutting grains and other processed stuffs out of your diet is very bad for the food industry? Remember that almost all the serious money to be made in the food sector is made through the sale of processed foodstuffs, not simple, fresh produce. Consider also how the pharmaceutical industry makes money out of patching up the ailments that processed foods cause. These neological foods actually keep both the food and drug manufacturers in business. Unfortunately, most doctors have a blind spot to this sort of information because they specialise in alleviating the symptoms of illness, not preventing them in the first place. The medical industry, like any other business, must remain profitable, and unfortunately, there is almost no money in preventative medicine – not when it consists of simply making sound food, exercise and lifestyle choices. Another impediment to getting the truth 'out there' is that there is precious little funding for scientific studies that aren't about justifying the sale of new, profitable drugs to the medical industry.

The proposition is this: human beings have not evolved to eat processed high-carbohydrate foods, nor can they eat many modern, manufactured foods without long-term harm.

In Chapter Two we outlined the host of modern diseases to which humans have only recently become prone. With every passing year the list of diseases – such as heart disease, IBS, Alzheimer's and arthritis – that revolve around the issue of increased inflammation and oxidisation of the organs and tissues grows longer.

Whatever is causing this damage is clearly rampant and out of control. So if at the end of this chapter you think that grain consumption and other modern toxins aren't the cause of all this misery, please let me know the better explanation you've come across. I beg you not to dismiss this chapter out of hand because of any short term 'inconvenience' its implications might cause you.

Want proof?

Why not give our 30 Day Challenge a try and see if you feel the difference yourself without grains in your diet? Visit www.instinctive–fitness.com for our 30-Day Challenge workbook.

You owe it to yourself (and those who are around you) to try some of these ideas and see for yourself if they make a difference. I intend to persuade you with logic initially, but ultimately I beg you to experiment with your own diet and find what works for you. Luckily, most people who make these changes are able to see and feel the changes reasonably quickly. There's just no need for blind faith.

If you commit to making a few simple changes for just a few weeks with the 30-day programme, I am confident that you will see enough of a difference to want to stick with it over the long term. Sure, it's not an overnight fix, but it will provide consistent workable results with a methodology you can stick to for the rest of your life. I assure you that the benefits will only continue to grow with passing time.

Are you ready for your 30-Day Challenge?

If you cut modern foods out of your life for at least a month, I guarantee you'll notice all or some of the following improvements:

*Less addiction to food (though you'll still enjoy it) * More consistent energy through the day * No after-meal energy lag * More resistance to cough, colds, flu, etc. * Weight loss of at least five pounds (which will continue until you reach your ideal body weight) * Clearer skin with fewer red patches and fewer allergic reactions * A reduced waist-line (this sometimes happens independently of weight loss) * An ability to miss meals without a feeling of weakness or desperation * Less dependence on stimulants like coffee to stay awake and to maintain your mood.*

Before you decide to accept or decline my little challenge, I'd like to outline why taking these steps is the ONLY acceptable approach to improved health.

The first reason is simple – through the eyes of evolution, all diets are, to a greater or lesser extent, a fad. Think about it. In terms of the millennia we've lived on this small, blue, spinning planet – almost everybody in the western world is today on a fad diet of one kind or another. Even if you just eat 'whatever', or the 'standard' British diet, or just whatever your partner puts in the fridge, you are still partaking in an entirely new experiment. All diets based around modern food are, through the long-seeing eyes of history, faddish; a mere flash in the pan.

You just need to look at the decline in the western world's health over the last 100 or so years to see its diet must be a 'fad'.

The diet of those in the 'developed' west

The diet that most of us in the west now eat is fairly easy to describe. It is broadly similar to the one the British Government advises us eat. That is to say, 'a balanced diet based around healthy grains, vegetables, and low in fat.' And this awful advice is where it all goes wrong.

A deadly harvest

As we discussed earlier, it was a just 10,000 years ago (a mere blink of an eye in evolutionary terms) that humans came up with a cunning new way to grow, harvest and mill grains and make them appear outwardly consumable. At the time they thought they were onto a winner with this more reliable source of food, but their nutrition problems were not over, but in fact only just beginning. Their health now depended, not on their supply of foraged food, or their hunting skills, but on how successful they were at neutralizing the toxins in a crop naturally resistant to consumption. They were now shackled to a laborious and time-consuming process involving grinding, soaking and cooking rather than a short-ish daily hunt and forage.

10,000 years ago, life undoubtedly got harder for the early farmers, but that wasn't the end of the story of mankind's decline. The grains we consume today bear little resemblance to those eaten only a few centuries grown and are now processed on an industrial scale. Today there are more than 25,000 species of grain, most of which we created in a laboratory to be disease resistant or produce high yields – *not* to be more nutritious. (For comparison, in Jesus's time there were only three – but I bet they were all much higher in essential vitamins.)

In order to achieve these profit-saving traits, scientists had to enhance the part of the grains that naturally resists disease and predators – mainly, gluten, lectins, and phytates – the most harmful parts of the grains to humans.

Following World War II, plant breeders developed new strains of grain that delivered higher yields with the intensive applications of nasty substances, such as artificial nitrogen, herbicides and pesticides. (These hybridized strains, sprayed with these filthy chemicals, are at least partly responsible for the growing number of allergies from which we suffer today.)

Because they wanted bigger yields and bigger profits, bakers called upon plant breeder to concoct crops with even more stretchy protein molecules to make their new, 'lighter' loaves. These new crops contained greater amounts of gluten, the protein molecule found in abundance in wheat, rye and other grains. This change seriously reduced the density of vital minerals and vitamins in the grain to offset the higher gluten content. Consequently, modern wheat strains are 30 to 40 per cent poorer in minerals such as iron, zinc and magnesium than the wheat eaten in the first half of the last century.

Here in modern day, industrial Britain, wheat is the crop of choice, found in pretty much every bread, cereal, biscuit and pasta. It's relatively cheap and we consume it by the skip-load. Of all the grains (including rye, barley and corn), wheat is the most popular and abundant. Unfortunately it's also the most harmful. Studies suggest that about two thirds of the UK population start their day with some form of cereal or bread. In doing so, these individuals start each day with something partially poisonous to them and a product devoid of most of the vitamins and minerals their body requires. Worryingly, the majority of the British population's calories come from just this one harmful grain.

It's an undisputed medical fact that some people are unable to consume any bread, or anything made of most grains because of the presence of **gluten** and other proteins. You'll probably have seen a growing number of gluten-free products in the shops, which allow celiac sufferers who have intestinal problems and cannot handle gluten to eat the same sort of products as the rest of us with apparent impunity. However, the obvious up-front symptoms that celiacs suffer from when they consume gluten are just the visible tip of a much bigger, wheat-shaped iceberg. Celiacs are just the small part of society who manifest their symptoms *immediately* and *obviously*. The rest of us still suffer the effects too – just quietly and on a time delay of years rather than hours, building up problems over the course of a lifetime.

But it's not just the gluten in the wheat that cause us problems either; oh no, it is the rest of the product as well. Like all grains, wheat contains a whole host of other defence mechanisms and, unlike a grass, which 'wishes' to be eaten by animals to disperse its seeds, a grain 'wishes' to repel animals from consuming it. To do so, it produces other antinutrients alongside gluten, such as lectins and phytates, which actually damage the digestive tracts of any animal that tries to eat it. That is why these noxious crops have survived for so many millennia and early humans were not daft enough to attempt to eat them.

These phytates (nasty little critters) actually stop the proper absorption of calcium, magnesium, copper, iron and zinc in the digestive tract – all of which are needed for good health[1]. The single fact alone explains a great deal of modern health issues. Google "mineral deficiency symptoms" if you're unsure of this. The list is long and painful to read.

To put it into context, no wild animals need to be told this information. There are none that choose to consume grain; their instinct tells them it's harmful to them. The only animals that do eat it are domesticated animals, which have no choice but be fed cooked grain in order to fatten them up. Ask any pig farmer.

Furthermore scientists now agree that proteins in grains, especially gluten, are *very* hard to digest. Modern, processed grains (whether 'wholemeal' or not) put an enormous strain on the entire digestive system.

A very modern, fluffy, white loaf

Along with most cereal, bread is one of the worst things that we can eat. One of the main problems is that our modern breads are baked to be light and fluffy, and they are almost all universally awful in their ingredients. There isn't really much difference, nutritionally speaking, between white and brown bread, despite the advertising propaganda. A better distinction is between the heavy, grainy, dense loaf of centuries gone and the attractive, addictive, junk food that passes for a bloomer, bap or baguette today.

Modern bread is a very different thing entirely to what Chaucer knew in the Middle Ages, and a substantially different product when compared to the bread your grandmother ate as a child. Her daily loaf would have contained much less gluten and more fibre. It also didn't instantly turn to sugar as soon as it reached her stomach – and it even had *some* beneficial nutrients floating around in it.

"The health of nations is more important than the wealth of nations."
Will Durant

It was only in the 1960s when bread took a *really* serious turn for the worse when a new development (the 'Chorleywood Process') meant that loaves could be produced more cheaply without having to wait the best part of a day for the yeast to ripen and rise.

Traditional methods of baking used to allow time for the dough to ripen and, in doing so, neutralise some of the wheat protein most likely to trigger bowel disease and other autoimmune and inflammatory conditions. In the greedy rush toward better productivity, modern bread producing methods don't do this at all, and so this bread presents an even more serious challenge for the body to metabolise properly.

Because these new breads were being made so quickly, there was no longer sufficient time given to ripening the dough, a process that makes it easier to handle and ensures it tastes good. In order to solve this problem, modern bread manufacturers use literally hundreds of additives to achieve these effects artificially.

These bread additives are derived from substances that no human would normally eat, but we were told they were safe until, one-by-one, scientists told us, actually, they weren't.

Almost at the point of despair, the industry found a new category of 'improvers' – additives based on industrial enzymes. These 'natural' sources of biological catalysts, obtained from cereals, mould, bacteria and even animal guts, now routinely go into bread.

Today, enzymes are the dirty little secret the baking industry is very reluctant to talk about.

This is what a modern 'wholemeal' loaf contains: *Wholemeal Flour, Water, Caramelised Sugar, Yeast, Fermented Wheat Flour, Salt, Vegetable Fat, Wheat Protein, Emulsifiers: E472e, E471, Soya Flour, Flour Treatment Agent: Ascorbic Acid* (source: the back of any bag of bread).

In fact the ingredients listed above aren't the whole 'roll' call by any means. The list of additives is so long and scary that the bread industry has been given special dispensation to simply use the terms 'flour treatment agents' and 'emulsifiers' to cover their tracks and not to risk ruining a whole 'slice' of the economy. The products get even worse when sugar, salt, soya, preservatives (e-numbers) and vegetable oil are added to the mix. You can see why we should no longer describe bread, as the Bible does, as the "staff of life".

All high-carbohydrate foods will mess you up

When it comes to grain, wheat-based bread and cereal is just the most delinquent example of a bad bunch. It is low-nutrient, high-carb, high-sugar and highly-additive products like this that you need to avoid if you want to recapture the energy, health and vitality you should enjoy naturally.

Although not *all* high-carb foods are intrinsically unhealthy, if you hope to lose weight you still probably want to avoid them for a while. Here's why:

1. *You probably can't handle even relatively healthy, starchy carbohydrates such as sweet potato or rice until you have repaired the damage the rest of the unhealthy carbs have done.*

2. *High-carb foods produce a sugar (glucose) rush to the bloodstream that the body fails to stabilise well. A failure to stabilise blood-glucose levels leads to an increased release of a hormone called* **insulin.**

3. *Insulin, a natural hormone, takes sugar out of your bloodstream and puts it into the muscles, but in the presence of too much high-carb fare (and too much sugar) it can't do its job properly. More and more insulin is required to complete the job as your body starts to resist its action. This is the start of* **insulin resistance***, a state most of us are in and which exists as a halfway house between good health and full-blown* **type II diabetes.**

4. *Increased levels of insulin tell the body to* **store fat***.*

In short, regular ingestion of most high-carb foods like pasta, potatoes and cereal will sooner or later make you obese, unable to handle sugar well, and incapable of metabolising fat properly as an energy source. It may also, given a little more time, give you diabetes. Sometimes, it gives you diabetes *before* it makes you fat – if you're really unlucky.

Overweight people looking to lose fat usually fall at the first hurdle. Ironically, individuals with faulty carbohydrate metabolisms are told by doctors, government officials and dieticians to eat *more* carbohydrates and *less* fat. In doing, so they make the damage worse and hasten their path towards toward obesity, insulin resistance and ill-health.

> The western diet is dominated by over-processed, high-carb, high-sugar, packaged 'bait food' peddled by the big corporations. It is food that is in fact designed specifically to hook you by your poor confused instincts straight to the checkout

This is the sad, mad, crazy road we have been travelling in the UK for decades.

Your body is hard-wired to turn excess carbs into fat

As a modern day hunter-gatherer, your body is hardwired to turn excess carbohydrate into fat. When it notices an increase in carb consumption it assumes that there is an absence of healthy calories around.

"Where is the meat? Where's the fat? Where's the protein?" it asks, hungrily.

Believing itself to be starved of good nutrition it assumes there is an impending famine and starts to frantically store any extra calories it can find as fat around the waist, bum and thighs.

This neat evolutionary adaptation meant that when our ancestors did not have access to as many calories as their bodies required, they could still use their stored body fat as their main source of sustained energy. Any fat around the body was easily broken down and used to supply calorific needs.

Ancient taste buds

What tasted best *was* best for our ancient ancestors. Our craving for fat, sweet and salty flavours today is no unfortunate coincidence – it's these very deep cravings (like sex) that kept our species going for millennia in an ancient world.

Stone Age man's palette was highly sensitised to the merest hint of sweetness or saltiness and was 'hard-wired' to seek it out, as this was his best indicator that a food would be high in fat and protein or essential nutrients. These preferences would encourage him to hunt and consume meat whenever possible, or certain sweet fruits, vegetables or honey. (Before we started cultivating them, most vegetables were, although more nutritious, saddled with a sourer taste than we are familiar with today.)

His love for sweet, salty or fatty foods discouraged him from choosing blander, less nutritional options like ground roots unless he had no other option. Given a choice between, say, bison and yams your body wants you to eat bison. As bison meat is, pound for pound, more nutritious than yams, it's no accident that in taste comparison tests, bison wins every time.

This drive for salty, sweet or fatty foods ensured our appetite remained fired up and able to motivate our behaviour towards hunting out our next nutritious meal.

Our sweet tooth once made us crave seasonal fruit or extremely limited supplies of honey. These were prized because of their nutritional value and, of course, their scarcity. These once rare and precious foods are now supplied year round by Tesco and other loveable supermarket chains, but the convenience of purchasing fruit and honey from middle-ranking supermarkets in itself isn't really the problem.

The real issue today is that modern foods are in fact imposters. These pseudo-foods are cunningly designed to mimic the tastes that we associate with healthy foods, while actually supplying us with something entirely different. They are a chimera, a poison chalice, a Trojan horse – use whatever metaphor you will.

Take breakfast cereal for example – any major brand. Even the ones that aren't 'frosted' (covered in cheap sugar) affect our bodies in the way that no component of a Paleolithic diet ever could.

The very moment the product enters our mouths it starts to break down and be digested very quickly (so quickly it might as well be pure sugar), and our taste buds are delighted they've been given something rare and sweet to feast on. Driven by the very oldest part of our brain, our instincts tell us that sweet things are special and should be eaten quickly while they're available. Of course we don't actually 'think' this, our body just *knows* this because it tastes so good, and leaves the conscious brain in peace to watch breakfast TV.

There isn't really anything like this in the wild. Fruit and honey are certainly sweet and do contain carbs, but they also contain nutrients and other goodies needed to stay healthy. More importantly they're also a 'here today, gone tomorrow' kind of thing in the wild – not something to depend on year round. Unfortunately, modern grains and cereal are much, much higher in carbohydrates, lower in every other form of nutrient and *are* readily available any time you want, year round.

The insulin trap

Modern, refined carbs are available for twelve months of the year and are rarely treated like an occasional indulgence. Cereals, grains and pasta form the rock bed of many people's diets. They break down almost instantly in the mouth and cause a massive rise the hormone, insulin. Insulin takes the sugar deposited in the bloodstream in the form of glucose out of the bloodstream and delivers it to the muscles where it can be used as energy. However, the body just isn't built to handle this much sugar this fast (as nothing exists like it in nature) so it demands more insulin to be produced than was ever intended to clear up all the sugar sloshing about in the system.

In a diet filled with this sort of high-calorie carbohydrate, the body is flooded with insulin on a long-term basis. Over time the muscles, reacting to the insulin, start to become de-sensitised and ignore the very important message it brings, and so stop taking this glucose into the muscles. This energy has got to go somewhere, so instead it is diverted and stored as fat.

The continual presence of all this sugar in the bloodstream raises blood glucose levels unnaturally high. The body is actually threatened by this and reacts by releasing adrenaline, giving the owner a temporary high.

However, everyone knows that what goes up must come down, so when the individual finally takes a break from this cereal-fest, their blood glucose levels crash, leading to instant fatigue, lethargy, premature sleepiness and sometimes depression (as with me in the bad old days). This is prime fat storing time.

Nobody likes feeling like this. Just like a junkie deprived of a hit, the body starts to crave another shot of adrenaline. *"Just one more hit, I can handle it,"* you lie to yourself, your appetite for sweet foods now thoroughly whetted. Later, you whine: "I'm so tired! Another bowl of cereal will give me the energy I need. After all, I felt on top of the world after the last one..." Our false reasoning only deepens the nutritional trap in which we have been so cleverly ensnared.

Boosted by our unrestrained instinct for more sweetness, we start the processed sugar hit and crash cycle all over again: reaching for more food that our bodies continue to mistake for the occasional treat that nature offers us.

Naughty carbohydrates!

As we've seen, taken to its furthest medical extreme, this process of carb craving and crashing is responsible for diabetes: a state where the body is no longer able to produce insulin to control blood glucose levels at all. If not injected with a man-made insulin substitute, the glucose eventually builds up and crystallises in the blood doing irreparable damage to the circulatory system.

The elephant in the room here that no one seems to want to talk about is the fact that *the real cause of Type I and Type II diabetes and obesity is the abuse of modern processed carbohydrates.*

Most adults have lost the ability to switch to burning stored fat; instead they run permanently on sugar (from sugar and carbs) in a way in which they were never 'designed' to.

On a personal note, I realised that I was getting skinny-fat when I was in my early thirties. Finally, I made the high-carb connection and stopped eating what is often called 'peasant food' – pizza, pasta, bread, cakes, rice, potatoes and biscuits. (In the Middle Ages bread was used as plates; no self-respecting king or landed gentry would be seen eating grains over meat).

In particular, I started avoiding gluten and stuck to meat, fish, vegetables, fruit and nuts. Very quickly two things happened. I lost all the fat around my waist that had been building up over the previous four or five years and, amazingly, I discovered I was no longer tired or depressed after meals. Previously I had found that after most meals I felt like lying down to sleep for a few hours. I assumed I was eating too much. Because sleeping was often inconvenient, I also became addicted to coffee to keep me going through the day.

After changing my diet I found that I could even eat large lunches and head into the afternoon full of energy. In fact, I had consistently high levels of energy through the day. These days I know myself well enough to remember that if I opt for even a single sandwich, my body will protest and I will feel like heading to the sofa.

Interestingly, even when I knew that bread, pizza and the like were messing me up, I still craved them. It took me a while to realise that I was actually addicted to the sugar rush they produced. The adrenaline rush I so enjoyed was caused by my body's attempt to handle what it recognised as a threat. I just wish that I had understood what was going on in my body a little sooner.

Many of my clients tell me they couldn't go back to eating grains – wheat in particular – even if they wanted to. They say that it makes them feel so grotty now that it just isn't worth it.

It seems that when we are consuming something regularly, even if it's bad for us, our bodies try to reduce our awareness of the symptoms; however, when we resume a harmful habit after a break from it, our body complains like never before in the hope of averting a return to previous bad habits.

Perhaps our bodies aren't as passive in our lives as we may have thought – and as we get healthier, we get more sensitive to unhealthy foods, not more able to tolerate them.

Friendly fat

Fat, however, is the perfect fuel for us. If it weren't, why would we store it around our bodies rather than starch or sugar? It is there because evolution decided it was the very best fuel to burn during lean times.

Fat does contain more calories per gram than carbohydrate, which goes someway to explaining its bad rap – but it satisfies our appetite much faster and for longer. Fat satiates the body largely because it is finally giving the body what it really needs. This is why when people eat more fat they invariably end up consuming *fewer* calories without even trying.

What people who have a phobia of body fat forget is that it is part of their body's grand design. It evolved this way for a reason. Body fat doesn't just mean we've done something dumb or greedy. *It's our body's defence against starving.* Our bodies evolved the ability to put fat into cells for a reason – to store energy, which is fine. The issue is that many of us have too much of it, and have lost the ability to re-metablise it once it has been stored away.

The problem is that so many of us are simply too messed up with a high carbohydrate intake to use our prime energy system. We don't consume much fat and we don't burn much of it. We're like a hybrid car that's stuck in one mode. Sedentary living, modern food toxins, too much stress and not enough sleep all exacerbate the problem. This general malaise and the long list of symptoms that accompany this overall lack of 'wellness' have led to the coining of terms such as 'Metabolic Syndrome' or 'Syndrome X'. These loose descriptions are used to describe an intangible feeling of dis-ease that GPs find it so hard to pin down. This is so because it can affect almost any part of your body at a cellular level and expresses itself in a bewildering range of unpleasant ways.

Choosing animal fat as your primary fuel though, means you are returning to your intended ancestral fuel source. And the best way to switch your metabolism into fat burning mode is to start eating more meat, eggs, fish and vegetables – and whatever (natural) fats comes with these.

You will come across people who'll try to throw you off-track by telling you that they eat cheesecake every meal or McDonald's twice a day and still weigh the same as they did in college. And maybe they do. Maybe they've been lucky enough to get away without significant damage so far. Or maybe they manage to run excess weight off with hours of cardio every week. Maybe they actually haven't been so lucky; it's just not that plain to see yet. Not all poor health is visible around the waist. Wait twenty years and check back with them. The older someone gets, the more seriously you can take the evidence of their health claims.

Fat – the good, the bad and the downright ugly

For decades now we have been bombarded with misinformation. We've been told repeatedly until our ears bleed that animal fat (which is high in fat, much of it saturated) is BAD and that vegetable oils (polyunsaturated fats/oils) are GOOD. So for decades now we have dutifully been spreading bland margarine rather than rich tasting butter on our morning toast, and cooking with vegetable oil rather than lard.

The fat situation is far more complicated than we've been led to believe.

"Sat Fat" Fears

The pop science explanation of the 'dangers' of saturated fat goes something like this:

"Y'see, when you eat fatty foods, especially those rich in animal fat, the saturated fat and cholesterol in these foods wind up in your blood and stick to your arteries. 'Cos saturated fats are solid outside your body, they will be solid inside your body too *(er, despite the 30-degree increase in average temperature?).* Arteries are much like pipes. When they get caked up with grease, blood flow is impaired, and a heart attack ensues."

This simple, primary-school-level explanation has caught hold of the public's imagination because it's so easy to understand with its 'think-about-why-your-sink-gets-blocked' analogy. It is, however, absolute nonsense. Not even the early scientists who set this anti-sat-fat train rolling had a notion of human biology that was this fundamentally wrong. Their explanation, although also incorrect, was at least partially logical and valid, unlike the popular notions that have stopped most people enjoying a substance that our bodies evolved to use as their major fuel.

Even mothers' breast milk is 50% fat, much of it saturated. Any biologist can tell you that saturated fat and dietary cholesterol are *essential* to a baby's growth.

However, we are told to believe that it somehow becomes deadly as we get older. Does that make sense to you?

To keep it simple and even remotely understandable, let's forget about all the confusion of **saturated fats (fats that are solid at room temperature) and unsaturated fats (fats that are liquid at room**

182

temperature); let's also put aside monounsaturated fats and polyunsaturated fats as well for the moment. Let's instead just look at fats from a common sense point of view, through the eyes of evolution.

Why caveman didn't fry their chips in vegetable oil (Not that they had potatoes...)

Before the days of factory-sized food refineries that crush, squeeze, heat and chemically strip the very last drop of fatty oil from vegetable seeds, ancient humans would have had only one significant source of fat: animal fat. This would have been prized as their main source of calories, and conveniently it came together with all the protein and other types of nutrients and minerals their bodies also needed – all packaged in a convenient furry, feathered or fish-shaped box.

Animal fat was an abundant natural substance and would have been consumed in large quantities. Rather than stripping the finest cuts of lean meat from the carcass and leaving the rest, every last morsel of fat, hoofs, brains, eyeballs – the lot – would have been valued and consumed.

Where animal fat would have been consumed by the fistful, vegetable oils (naturally occurring in vegetable seeds) would have been merely a trace element in our diet. This was due, firstly, to the tiny amount of oil contained in the seeds, and secondly, seeds just weren't available in the vast quantities we see in today's intensively farmed world.[5]

Ancient man would have consumed large quantities of animal fat but vegetable fat only in infinitesimally small quantities.

Today, due to decades of scaremongering, we now shun these nutritious animal fats which sustained us perfectly for millions of years, and consume ridiculous amounts of highly processed vegetable oil we were never designed to eat, in the form of margarines, bread, cakes and other processed foods.

It is my hope that, where before you read this chapter you would have gone to the kitchen cupboard and happily taken out a 'golden bottle of nutritious, vegetable goodness', you will come to see vegetable oil for what it really is. **Mary Enig**, author of *Know Your Fats : The Complete Primer for Understanding the Nutrition of Fats, Oils and Cholesterol* describes this sort of stuff as:

"...a totally unnatural, dangerous, relatively indigestible 'plastic.'"

183

Fats matter

Even though the mere mention of the word 'fat' strikes fear into most of the population, fats (shortened from 'essential fatty acids') are truly *essential* to normal body function. They are the "active ingredient" in every bodily process including:

- *brain cell function and nervous system activity*
- *hormones and intra-cellular messengers*
- *glandular function and immune system operation*
- *haemoglobin oxygen-transport system*
- *cell wall function:*
    - *passing oxygen into the cell*
    - *passing nutrients into the cell*
    - *keeping foreign bodies out of the cell*
- *digestive-tract operation*
    - *assimilating nutrients*
    - *blocking out allergens*

This is true to the point that, arguably, essential fatty acids are *the* most important nutrients of all – more so than vitamins, minerals, or even proteins[2]. Because...

Without fats, there is no life.

So with fats being so essential to life itself, why have we come so petrified of the smallest morsel of fat passing our lips? It really makes no sense at all that the supposedly 'enlightened' western world has turned its back on it.

The main problem is we just don't eat much natural fat anymore: we shun animal fat and most of the vegetable-based oils we do consume have been chemically altered through a process called hydrogenation.

"The food you eat can either be the safest and most powerful form of medicine...or the slowest form of poison"
Ann Wigmore

What is hydrogenation?

Hydrogenation is the truly charming process of heating all types of vegetable seed oil up to structurally damaging temperatures and forcing hydrogen bubbles through it. The natural fatty acids in the oil then 'pick up' some of the introduced hydrogen, which has the effect of making the substance less viscous (runny) and therefore denser.

If the oil is 'fully hydrogenated', a solid fat type substance is created from the previously runny oil. But if the process is stopped part way through, a semi-solid *partially hydrogenated oil* with a consistency similar to butter is the result, only it's a whole lot cheaper (and nastier).

Previously, natural coconut oil had been used by food producers to create a rich, even texture in food. Nowadays however, they turn to partially hydrogenated fats with their artificially smooth, silky consistency and low cost, to create products with a similar feel for a greater profit.

Unfortunately hydrogenated fat is pretty much inedible and
fundamentally damaging.

What's wrong with hydrogenation?

Vegetable oils become monumentally nasty when hydrogenated[3] because they now contain high levels of **trans fats**: Their structure is altered at an atomic level and an otherwise normal fatty acid is "transmogrified" by high-heat processing. Nice!

These 'Frankenstein' fatty acids then have their atoms further messed about with by double-linking, cross-linking, bond-shifting, twisting and whole host of other exciting things that just serve to make them even more lethal.

Even though the sound of all this fiddling doesn't sound too appetising in itself, the real problem lies once this unnatural fatty substance gets into the body. The chemically active part has been messed up, but the "anchor end" (the part that attaches to the cell wall) is essentially unchanged. The body doesn't detect all the devious skulduggery that has gone on, so ushers these odious compounds to take up important positions somewhere in the body's cell walls. But like a drunken security guard, these modified atoms are totally incapable of doing their job properly – letting damaging foreign bodies pass right through, but stopping supplies of vital goodies from getting in.

Do you really want this hideous stuff in your body, stuff that has never before existed in our evolution and we've never had the need to evolve a defence against?

In the very unlikely event that you're still shrugging your shoulders and thinking 'so what' – you should know that this oil/fat hybrid is then literally steamed and perfumed to remove its foul odour. This stuff is actually rancid and would otherwise stink far worse than rotten meat or butter. Thanks to this final, sneaky process though, the consumer will never find out.

Trans fats will also make you fat

Research indicates that trans fats cause comparatively more weight gain than the same diet with monounsaturated fats and lead to a redistribution of body fat tissue to the abdominal area, the riskiest place to carry extra padding. Additionally, they're associated with inflammation and atherosclerosis, the processes responsible for cancers, heart conditions and most other modern diseases.

A 2004 study by Brigham and Women's Hospital and Harvard School of Public Health showed that in postmenopausal women, the more trans fats they ate and, to a much lesser extent, the more carbohydrate they ate, the worse their atherosclerosis (hardening of the arteries) became over time. Interestingly, the more saturated fat they ate, the less their atherosclerosis progressed; in the group with the highest intake of saturated fat, the atherosclerosis actually reversed over time.[4]

Trans fats are so bad that even the establishment has had to acknowledge their pernicious effects. In the states of New York and California they've been banned, while Denmark was the first country to ban them outright. It is hypothesised that the Danish government's efforts to decrease trans fat intake from six grams to one gram per day over 20 years is related to a 50% decrease in deaths from ischemic heart disease.[6]

Amazingly though, the UK food authorities appear to still be fine with their use. You can still find trans fats in half the products in your local supermarket. Typically they'll be found in margarine, bread, pastries, donuts, muffins, biscuits, cookies, cakes, pies, crackers, chips, instant-flavoured coffee drinks, microwave popcorn, and the usual fast food suspects like fried chicken and french fries. (N.B. 'shortening' is another term used for this awful stuff we would do well to avoid.)

If it's so bad, why do manufacturers use it? Well it's about profit again of course. Trans fats produce a crispy, flaky feel to food and extend it beyond its natural shelf life. Customers, unless they are biologists or nutritionists, have little idea what they are actually eating. Producers are forced by law to print this information on their labels, but I'm sure it hasn't missed your notice that they do a fine job of disguising the truth in the tiniest writing, ambiguous E numbers, and various other forms of devious sneakery.

Once you start reading labels, you'll realise that trans fats and vegetable oils are everywhere. So much mixed-ingredient food is contaminated with the stuff. The replacement of butter with margarine and vegetable oil has been one of the most harmful changes the west has made to its diet since we first walked out of the jungle.

So what can I use then?

Simple. Cook instead with:

- *Butter or ghee*

- *Tallow and suet from beef and lamb*

- *Lard from pigs*

- *Chicken, goose and duck fat*

- *Coconut, palm and palm kernel oils*

And for Salads:

- *Extra virgin olive oil*

Practically speaking then, this means cutting out all vegetable oils except coconut oil, olive oil and palm oil (none of which are made by crushing and processing seeds.) Specifically, do not eat or cook vegetable oil (sometimes referred to on labels as 'vegetable fat') made from the contents of highly processed seeds. Examples of these are sunflower, corn, safflower, cottonseed, peanut or soybean oil. Avoid these like the plague.

Of all the subjects covered in this book, undoubtedly the subject of fat consumption requires the biggest leap of both open-mindedness and faith.

Assuming you're under the age of 60, you will *never* remember a time when animal fat was officially 'OK' to eat. You will have had the 'animal fat is bad' message fired at you from every angle for a lifetime and will probably have heard this message of doom *millions* of times.

The greatest thinkers of the 15th century thought the world was flat, and that stars were pinholes that let the light of heaven shine through. In just the same way, in time, the last 60 years of fat advice will also be proven irrefutably to be wrong. The damage this brief folly has done to our health however is immeasurable and it's time for us to wake up to the truth.

Other non-foods

It's not just the high-carb, vegetable oils and trans fats that you need to look out for. The western diet is now filled with substances that shouldn't really be dignified with the description 'food'. Many of these can't be mentioned by name as they come in so many guises and under many brand names (and I don't like being sued). However they have certain things in common.

'Bait foods'

Think of a juicy worm wriggling on a hook, placed there to catch a fish. Fish are no intellectual giants and cannot help but take the bait that they are hard-wired to seek out. 'Bait Foods' are the equivalent for we hapless humans – products dressed up to hook our money using our poor, confused instincts. Their packaging and appearance are specifically designed to lure us in by mimicking the healthiest, nutrition-filled fruits and vegetables – and by being shinier, brighter and more colourful than any natural food. They are, in fact, neither healthy nor nutritious.

Bait foods usually:

- *have a long list of dodgy, sometimes unpronounceable ingredients.*

- *come packaged in fancy boxes.*

- *are pre-cooked (sometimes, not always).*

- *advertise spuriously dubious features (e.g. 'low-fat', 'added iron').*

- *are not actually a food (e.g. apple is a food; a crispy pancake is not – unless there's a pancake tree in nature that I'm unaware of...)*

- *have long, silly names (e.g. 'I-can't-believe-we-sell-this-stuff-instead-of-butter').*

Dodgy ingredients – Look out for packaged bait foods with:

- **Vegetable oil** – *The natural filler and lubricant of processed food everywhere. Nasty.*

- **Added sugar** – *Any additional sugar in your diet adds to the same problem as high-carbs – a swamping of the glucose energy system with instantly available energy, which leads to excess insulin, which leads to body fat retention. It also deranges your palate so that you can no longer enjoy the subtler taste of good food.*

- **Added salt** – *this is always in the form of table salt (sodium). Table salt has been stripped of all of the useful minerals that are found in natural rock salt or sea salt. An excess of this can affect your blood pressure.*

- **Added starches** – *e.g. cornstarch, tapioca starch, potato starch. These produce the same problems as grain consumption.*

- **Artificial colouring and flavouring** – *known as E numbers. You'll have read about the dangers of these before. They are implicated in conditions such as Attention Deficit Hyperactivity Disorder, and mood and behavioural disorders, especially in childhood.*

- **Artificial sweeteners** – *These have many names, such as: fructose, sucrose, dextrose, maltodextrin, aspartame – even eating tablespoons of sugar is better than consuming these harmful alternatives. Fizzy drinks, sports drinks and most protein powders are rife with this stuff. All sugar substitutes other than stevia and xylitol are made from this unnatural stuff. The long-term effect of consumption is still a huge, dangerous unknown, but they are potentially carcinogenic according to some health researchers.*

- **Excess caffeine** – *A cup or two of organic coffee a day is ok, but heavily-caffeinated 'energy' drinks will disrupt your entire metabolism and hormonal balance. Excess caffeine can also be used to mask energy imbalances and disrupted blood glucose levels. Avoid.*

- **Soya** – *Is grain-like and contains **lectins, phytates and phytoestrogens**. The latter increase the production of the oestrogen hormone, producing 'moobs' in men. The quantities of this found in vegetarians' diets is just one more reason to avoid being one if you can.*

189

What the food companies really mean

1. *No added sugar – "Instead we've added a selection of sweet tasting, carcinogenic chemicals called artificial sweetener."*

2. *No artificial flavouring – "we've been kind enough not to add a concoction of chemicals will trick your brain into thinking you're eating something healthy."*

3. *Natural Flavouring – "a tiny drop of lemon has been added to the chemical crap we're already poisoning you with."*

4. *Low-fat – "We've taken the healthy fat out and replaced it with a horrible smorgasbord of industrially-processed food waste."*

5. *An essential source of vitamins and minerals – "We've added a tiny selection of manufactured vitamins back into a product whose nutritional benefits we've already stripped bare."*

By now you should be getting a pretty good idea of what, from an evolutionary point of view, is good to eat. Here is the Instinctive Fitness approach to eating:

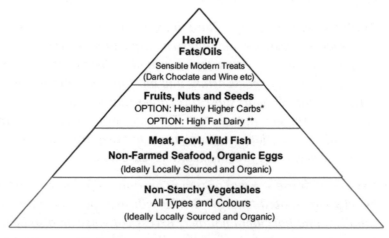

* e.g. sweet potato, wild rice, buckwheat – good, if not looking to lose weight
** Be sure to do a withdrawal test to ensure dairy works with your digestive system

The pyramid is arranged by recommended food *volume* (not calories, which would place meat, fowl, etc at the bottom instead of vegetables). The idea is that you eat more of those foods at the 'base' of the pyramid than those at the top.

There are lots – I mean hundreds – of alternative 'diets' out there that will take you seriously off track if you fall for their hype. Most diets today have been built upon the received wisdom of accepted nutritional science (low-fat, high-carb), so they try in vain to twist the plain facts into 'new', more palatable and marketable models. As soon as you move away from the principle that we should eat what we evolved to eat, any nutrition advice becomes increasingly hard to justify.

Here is a very brief overview of the main 'wonder' diets that have appeared recently:

Low-fat diets

I think we've dealt with this already. Low-fat means that to get the calories your body needs, you must turn to extra grain and heavy-carbs as an alternative source of calories. It also usually means processed instant meals with nasty ingredients.

Low-calorie diets

Leaping into bed with the government's low-fat advice is the super-low-calorie approach to weight loss. If you remember though, our bodies have been programmed by evolution to try to hang onto fat when threatened by the possibility of running short of nutrients or fat to burn. When you cut the calories, your body feels threatened and will try to retain the fat it already has. Instead, the weight you lose (if any) will be in the form of excess water (we're made of 60% water of course) and depleted muscle mass.

Weightwatchers® is the classic example of this. This multi-national company founded its credentials on the idea that eating fewer kilocalories of energy by sticking to Weightwatchers® 'low-fat' meals is a great way to lose weight. It's low calorie by dint of the fact they're low in fat, but they are usually high in sugar and low in essential nutrients.

Sticking with the Weightwatchers® plan (and it's not easy) means you will likely lose weight in the short-term but you will lose muscle as well as any fat. Muscle actually consumes calories during the day so, having lost muscle, the same number of calories you used to consume will make you fatter than you used to be as fewer calories will be consumed by your muscle mass. Since no one can eat like this for very long (long-term hunger hurts and is your body telling you something) you will inevitably go back to your old habits and put all the weight back on again – and more besides. If you're smart you might conclude that Weightwatchers® doesn't work; if you're not you will reason that things were fine when you were with on the programme, so you'll sign up for a few more months of misery.

This low-calorie/low-fat approach is *really* widespread now, despite the fact it clearly doesn't work. "Just eat less and exercise more," we are told by condescending, ignorant, overweight, hypocritical government ministers. If it were that simple, everybody could do it and nobody would need to write books about it.

There are no books, for example, about changing light bulbs, as far as I know. That's because it's relatively easy. There are loads of books about diets, because almost none of them work for people in the long term. 90% of them are variations of the idea of trying hard to eat less food/fat/calories – and fail to take account of the way that the body handles different sorts of foods, our nutritional requirements or our instinctive biological drives.

Vegetarianism/veganism

Gosh, this one's a real can of worms. Suffice to say that humans evolved to eat meat. There really isn't any serious debate about this, although you might start to doubt this if you stray onto a vegetarian website. Here you will read that we are actually so much like primates that we should still be eating fruit, as that's what apes eat. We should also eat vegetables and grains because apes also eat... Oh no, they don't do they? Well I'm not sure entirely how the argument hangs together. They also like to conveniently miss out the fact that chimpanzees, our nearest living evolutionary cousins, also eat meat in the form of smaller primates whenever the opportunity arises.

To be fair, vegetarianism can produce some good short-term results, such as if somebody opts for extra veg instead of eating the usual rounds of McDonald's, vegetable-oil-cooked, MSG-filled Chinese meals, pork pies and crisps. Pretty much everybody will start to feel better under those circumstances. The problem is that a vegetarian diet is not a safe, long-term option. It is simply too low in complete proteins and healthy fat sources, and alternatives to meat and fish are just not adequate to get the vitamins and nutrition we all need. *Beans are not a complete protein source* and do not supply a vegetarian with the healthy fats or vitamins they require either. For example a vegetarian would have to eat *39 eggs a day* to get the RDA (recommended daily amount) of Vitamin D (16mcg). Also, certain vitamins like A, D, E and K are fat-soluble. This means they can only be absorbed in the presence of fat, which the vegetarian diet rarely provides, unless huge quantities of eggs or diary are consumed. The result is an almost certainly deficiencies in the essential building blocks of good health – though it may take years for these problems to become apparent.

Vegetarians often end up eating huge quantities of tofu and soya, neither of which are healthy replacements.[7] They also have to consume a lot of grain and beans to keep hunger at bay. Vegetarians are usually weak and spindly or kind of fat; rarely do you see one with low-levels of fat and a reasonably healthy amount of muscle.

Paleo v vegetarian ethics

Some vegetarians will tell you that they have chosen their diet because the consumption of meat and dairy is unsustainable and can't be a staple for seven billion people. This seems to me a moot point, actually – and the subject for another book entirely. A better question is whether it makes sense to continue advocating a high-carbohydrate, high-grain diet when it has allowed the world's population to grow to a point where it seems it cannot be sustained with genuinely healthy foods.

Is the answer for everyone to continue to eat unhealthily so that the world's population can continue to grow ad infinitum?

However, this is all beside the point; the world as a whole still has massive surpluses in food supplies. The EU is paying large sums of hard cash to its farmers to *not* produce crops while other parts of the world starve. The reason that these parts of the world do not have enough to eat is because of politics and poverty – a failure to distribute resources adequately – not a lack of production *per se.*

As far as animal welfare goes, responsible Paleo eating involves choosing local produce that comes from well-treated animals, which have lived healthy, happy lives. Large-scale industrial farming is another thing entirely and should not be put in the same bracket.

Low GI diets

Having read the section on insulin, you'll probably understand how this is actually quite sensible. The GI (Glycaemic Index) is a measure of how quickly a carbohydrate-based food breaks down into glucose and enters the bloodstream. Bread, for example is given a rating of about 75, whereas sweet potato is given a rating of about 54. Both of these foods are carbohydrates, starchy and high in calories, but the sweet potato is the better choice because it will not produce the same elevated blood glucose levels (and corresponding insulin levels) that (nasty, modern) bread will.

The only criticism of the diet is that while it's okay for weight loss, it's not necessarily healthy. There are foods filled with grain and processed nastiness which, according to the numbers, should result in weight loss but actually won't as they cause an increased inflammatory response which is counter-productive for both weight loss and improved good health. For example, malt loaf is quite low in the GI index but can't be recommended for weight loss or better health.

The Atkins diet

Poor old, much-maligned Atkins. Say what you will about him, but it cannot be denied that people who followed his diet (a diet, if you believe what people say, consisting of nothing but meat and eggs) lost *a lot* of weight. Protein and fat is very satiating, so it's hardly surprising that people ended up eating fewer calories without really meaning to. Adherents also didn't lose too much muscle mass either (unlike turning vegetarian or going super-low calorie) as the higher protein diet provided all the building blocks they needed to maintain muscle mass.

His meat/egg/fish heavy diet was criticised by the establishment for eschewing 'healthy' carbs (like bread!) and encouraging the consumption of 'dangerously high' levels of saturated fat. When he contracted cardiomyopathy in 2000, a vegan group (with a drum to beat) put about a lot of false rumours that his heart condition was diet related. Some of the mainstream media were quick to use this as evidence of the unhealthiness of his diet.

In fact, his doctor said at the time that there was no evidence that his diet contributed to the condition. His cardiologist stated that (other than the cardiomyopathy) Atkins had "an extraordinarily healthy cardiovascular system". His coronary arteries were checked at that time and found to be free of blockages.

Much of what Atkins proposed was eminently sensible. He is sometimes criticised for not placing enough emphasis on the consumption of fresh vegetables, but even this may be a misrepresentation of the full

194

Atkins plan, which reinstated vegetables after only a few weeks of withdrawal. Unfortunately, in phases four and five, it also reinstated grains, had no concern about meat quality and allowed the consumption of vegetable oils and artificial sweeteners. Oh well, no one's perfect...

(Interestingly it seems that human beings *can* actually live on meat alone. Indeed, certain tribes, both ancient and modern, have done so for thousands of years. The Inuit, for example, as discussed earlier, live of a diet of almost nothing but saturated blubber from seals, whales, etcetera, year round. However, there is a caveat: to get all the nutrients, vitamins and minerals and anti-oxidants that a diet rich in vegetables would provide, you have to eat the *whole* animal – brains, liver, kidneys, bone marrow – everything. Not many of us are prepared to do this of course, so vegetables remain a tasty, nutritious and pretty much unavoidable component of a good diet.)

Fasting

"Fat people who want to reduce should take their exercise on an empty stomach and sit down to their food out of breath... Thin people who want to get fat should do exactly the opposite and never take exercise on an empty stomach".

Hippocrates

For thousands of years fasting has been an important, sometimes unavoidable part of people's lives, and certainly going without food occasionally was an inescapable fact of life for the hunter-gatherer. For many civilisations that followed, deliberate fasting was included as an established religious, social or health practice. Islam, Buddhism and Christianity all have their own stories and practices. There are probably multitudinous reasons for this, but in almost every culture, bar our own, fasting has been used as a gateway to superior emotional, spiritual or physical health. Did all these other cultures, independently, invent a pointless (not to mention challenging) practice – or is it just possible that they have something to teach the modern, western world?

We've already discussed the folly of low-calorie diets so you might think that fasting is merely an extreme version of the same and therefore to be dismissed. Surprisingly though, the science suggests that short periods of fasting can produce a great many benefits without the slower metabolism or muscle loss that long-term, low-calorie diets (and long-term fasting) can produce.

195

There may be no other culture that is as scared to deprive itself of food, even temporarily, than ours. Because so many of us run our bodies predominantly on carbs and sugar, we become afraid to miss even a single meal. If it does happen for any reason, it leaves us feeling lousy – tired, jittery, hungry and lightheaded – and just confirms in our minds the importance of eating at regular intervals. If however our diet consisted of more healthy fat and less carb, we would not find the occasions when we have to do without food to be particularly stressful at all.

Moreover, science has recently revealed that when the body experiences a noticeable reduction in calories it produces very specific changes in its chemistry.

By undertaking the occasional fast you will:

- *kick-start weight loss*

- *encourage anti-aging mechanisms*

- *reduce oxidation stress (it's a detox!)*

- *improve immune system defences*

- *stabilise blood-sugar levels and improve insulin sensitivity*

- *improve hormonal balances*

- *make your mind clearer and sharper*

You might wonder why this should be the case, and most conventional scientists cannot seem to adequately explain it. But perhaps an evolutionary standpoint may throw some light on a perplexing subject...

Our bodies are still optimized to survive in a world that is erratic in the supply of calories and nutrients.

Does it not make perfect sense that the body changes the way it operates when supplies of calories are scarce? To use an analogy: during an economic recession new house building drops and structural maintenance of properties goes up. In a similar way, does it sound so far-fetched that in times of hardship the body repairs and maintains cells rather than demolishing and replacing them?

It imperative that your body occasionally gets the signal that calories are in short supply so you can continue to thrive as an organism.

Your genes are pretty selfish: They care little about you, and only care about their own survival. When calories are abundant, your body concerns itself less with extending *your* longevity, as it will assume that your progeny will survive to pass on your genes.

Nasty genes

Scientists have been trying to find a magic formula for longevity for decades. However, in thousands of trials with mice, *only* calorie restriction has consistently been shown to extend average and maximum life spans – and it does so by between 30 to 50 per cent. What we've only just discovered is that these same benefits can be enjoyed by humans, even if they fast only for very short periods of time.

Perhaps one of the biggest gaps between our modern eating patterns and our evolutionary past and is the lack of variability in calories consumed from day to day. We evolved to eat as much as we could, just as often as we could – which was much of the time, *but not all the time*. Sometimes we would just *have* to go without, and perhaps the body has evolved to thrive with this 'boom and bust' model of eating that it just can't with a continual, monotonous supply of calories.

On occasion our ancestors would have hunted (exercised /walk/ sprinted) vigorously without success. They would have often exercised on an empty stomach – sometimes more than once before having the chance to consume significant calories again.

This meant that they became adapted to providing energy from stored body fat while maintaining steady blood glucose levels. Any fasted exercise they did forced them to dip into their fat reserves (hence there was always a serious absence of fat cavemen). By way of contrast, us modern folk have almost all been taught to 'fuel-up' before exercise. The result of this is that we must burn through glucose and glycogen supplies in the body before we can begin using any body fat as fuel. This is the simple reason that most people don't lose much weight even if they start an exercise programme. In fact, because they are unused to having low glucose levels in their blood, they will almost always eat more carbohydrate after exercise to make up for the increased hunger they experience. Hence regular exercisers can often get fatter.

Various protocols are currently being tested for their effects on health, weight and longevity. One possible approach is **Alternate Fasting**. This involves restricting every second day to about one third of normal calorie intake – say 500-700 calories. On the other day the faster is free to eat whatever and however much of whatever they want.

Another, perhaps easier, approach some people have experimented with is the 5-2 method. In any given week five days are spent eating normally to the point of satiation and two days are spent on a lower calorie intake, as above. The two days do not necessarily have to be consecutive.

Going back into the distant past it's reasonable to suppose that low-calorie fasts occurred on days when hunting had been unsuccessful and there wasn't any meat to go around. To try to make up the deficit ancient humans would probably have tried to consume as much fruit, veg and berries as possible. It would make sense therefore if on low-calorie fasting days we consume plenty of healthy vegetables, rather than emphasise meat or fish.

On days when fat and meat were simply not available, we would surely have resorted to plenty of easily digestible, healthy, anti-oxidants in the form of plant matter. This imposed healthy eating plan would have given the body an invaluable opportunity to clear its system while saving the body from the tougher metabolic task of breaking down protein, fat and the additional calories they contain. It would be an occasion for the body to go into "clean and filter" mode rather than the "build" mode it's in when it has access to proteins and fats.

In the "Putting It All Together" programme in Chapter Twelve it's suggested that you deliberately miss a meal or two each week to disrupt the usual 3-or-more-meals-a-day (plus snacks) routine that most of us fall into. You could consider this a good starting point. If you are more ambitious or experimental than this then there is much potential for fasting to be used to even greater effect. The 5-2 method might be a very good place to start.

You'll realise by now that what is being proposed is not so much a diet as an eating style, focusing on **what** to eat. In terms of body composition (or just 'looking great naked', if you prefer), *eating the right foods is 80% of the battle.* It really doesn't matter if you are an aspiring bodybuilder, want to look like Bruce Lee or Megan Fox, or just want to lose that paunch – it really is all about the food.

That said, please avoid becoming totally hung up on eating. Counting every calorie, measuring your food, or weighing yourself daily is borderline neurotic behaviour.

No self-respecting cavemen ever weighed themselves!

The plan should be dead simple. Here it is:

- *Start by eliminating all the offensive, processed food, grains, sugar and industrial oils*

- *Eat meat, seafood, eggs, vegetables, fruit, nuts, herbs and spices and healthy oils*

- *Eat two or three times a day – no more*

- *Vary calorific intake from day-to-day*

- *Don't skimp on high quality foods*

Choosing good food

Every bit of extra income you spend on improving the quality of your food is the best investment in your future you can make.

Meat

Go for organic and/or local meats whose flesh comes from animals free from injected growth hormones, antibiotics and other stimulants. Choose anything from beef, pork, lamb, chicken, venison, quail, duck, turkey, and other whole meat products. Wild game is great. Salami, spam and processed ham are out. Liver, kidneys and other organ meat are superlative and contain certain vitamins that are hard to get elsewhere. Organic bacon is wonderful and, now you've got over your 'sat-fat' fears, can be demolished without guilt at your leisure.

Endeavor to buy beef (or whatever) that is **100% grass-fed** ('pasture fed'). I can't emphasise this enough. Cows should eat grass, not grain. Many people remain blissfully unaware that animals are often reared on industrial feeds they would *never* eat in the wild. For example, the most modern, intensive, industrial farms rear cows housed in giant barns all-year-round where they consume a concentrated diet of corn, grain and soy.

Because of their cramped living conditions and unnatural diet, they have to be force-fed large quantities of antibiotics. These are used routinely to prevent mastitis, an infection of the udder, which occurs much more frequently in animals that are intensively milked. As a result of consuming meat from animals that have been injected like this, British people are becoming increasingly resistant to strains of potentially life-saving antibiotics. As our farming practises rush headlong in the direction of the USA in search of profitability (where farming is *highly* intensive and hormones are permitted to fatten cattle quicker) we will have to become even more wary of the provenance of the meat we eat.

Buy meat produced locally. Even if you're not interested in the ecological arguments (transportation costs, fuel consumption, air pollution, etc.) or the ethical arguments (about inhumane travelling conditions for animals), the fact is that local food arrives in a much fitter state for consumption than that which comes from the other side of the country or the other side of the world. Animals that have been well-treated have much lower levels of stress hormones, and that improves the quality of their meat considerably.

Supermarkets sell food that is a lot older than you might like to think, and by the time you consume it, it has only a fraction of the nutrients it would have had when fresh.

Look into local suppliers, ideally straight from a local farm. *www. bigbarn.co.uk* will give you some idea where to start if you want to take this road.

Many people think it's kinder to give their custom to farms that keep their animals outside for most of the year rather those that house them on top of each other in enormous barns where they have no contact with nature and little room to move.

Fish and Seafood

Choose wild fish, never fish that has been farmed. Farmed fish comes laced with dioxins, (cancer-linked) PCBs, fire retardants , pesticides (especially for sea lice), antibiotics, copper sulphate (to take care of algae on the nets), and canthaxanthin (a dye to make grey farmed fish various shades of "wild" pink). If you do eat farmed fish, environmental groups suggest you eat no more than one serving per month. That tells you all you need to know about farmed fish.

Eggs

Choose local free-range eggs, of course. Ideally 'pasture fed' and organic. Don't sponsor the madness that keeps hens shut up in tiny cages for their whole lives. Even if you don't care about this, the lower quality of egg is more than enough reason to avoid eggs from caged-hens.

You should look for chickens that have a chance to get outside during the day and, ideally, forage for their own food. It is okay if they have been fed some grain as chickens (unlike cattle) have a digestive system that is properly equipped to process the stuff. However, chickens are actually omnivores and are at their very best when digging around for bugs, worms and other bits of protein. If you can buy poultry and eggs from someone who keeps their chickens like this, you're doing really well.

Free-range is almost a given these days amongst thinking people who aren't on the breadline (a well-chosen phrase, as I'd have to be desperate before I bought supermarket bread). However many people who wouldn't ever dream of buying anything other than 'free-range' eggs quite innocently consume plenty of the battery-farmed variety in the processed foods they buy. Oh, the irony.

Vegetables

Eat lots of them. They should fill up more than half the space on your plate. Choose lots of different coloured vegetables (as silly as that sounds) as the different colours denote different types of vitamins and anti-oxidants. "Eat the rainbow, man" – as they say in the USA. Due to their nutritional profile, green vegetables (spinach, broccoli, kale, lettuce, seaweed, etc.) are of particular importance.

Potatoes are, of course, also a vegetable, but they were bred to be extra starchy in the New World. They won't help in weight loss and don't offer much in terms of good nutrition. When you reach your ideal 'fighting weight', and you have moved away from being a perennial, sugar-burning 'carb-head', you might consider including them again if you are exercising pretty hard.

Vegetables are where you are going to pick up many of the vitamins you need to live healthily, to keep a strong immune system, and to delay the on-set of premature ageing. This is the secret hidden in plain view. Buying **organic** not only avoids contaminants from the farming process, but also produces a product that is richer in nutrients than those grown in our increasingly mineral-depleted soils.

If you're hoping for a 'miracle' recovery from serious disease, you could start by looking at nine portions of vegetables a day. Watch **Dr. Terry Wahls** in "Minding Your Mitochondria" on YouTube for an eye-opening personal account of the power of vegetables.

Again ideally buy *local, organic vegetables* that will be far fresher and freer from contaminants, pesticides and herbicides.

Fruits

Fruit is great in moderation and eaten whole. Some confer the same amazing health-giving properties as vegetables. As with vegetables, try to choose local and organic (or at least wash them thoroughly).

Fruits are, however, heavier on sugar, and modern fruit is not quite the same products as those our forest-dwelling ancestors would have eaten. Early fruit, pre-cultivation, would have been more sour and fibrous. This only starts to make a measurable difference if you start chugging fruit juices by the carton or eating one banana after another. (Bananas are quite carb heavy – beware).

If you must drink fruit juice then ensure it is not 'from concentrate' and dilute it with water as much as is palatable. Remember it's usually the skin of fruit that's rich in nutrients rather than the juice, which contains mostly sugar (fructose). Avoid dried fruits because they're *very* sugary and often glazed in vegetable oil.

Nuts

A bit like fruit: great in moderation. There's no doubt they are a healthy, natural food, filled with B vitamins and essential minerals like magnesium, calcium, potassium, zinc and iron. If you've eaten a small handful to reach a meal to avoid your still-stabilising blood glucose levels dropping too low, that's fine.

If you are necking them by the pocketful every day, you are going to be consuming a lot of very dense calories, which may seriously impede weight loss. Also make sure they are not coated in sugar or vegetable oil. The best nut is the macadamia; these are so packed full with nutrients they can almost be considered a super food. By the way, despite their misleading name, peanuts are not a nut; they are a legume in disguise – avoid.

Salad oils and cooking oils

Use virgin, cold-pressed olive oil for salad dressing. Avoid vegetable oil made from superheated (hydrogenated) seeds. Cook meat and vegetables with any sort of animal fat, butter or ghee. Goose or duck fat is great, as is coconut oil. Avoid heating olive oil up much as it degrades in the same way as mass-produced, rancid, dangerous vegetables oils that are damaged in the hydrogenation process. Store it at room temperature in the dark. *Remember that fat is needed for the body to absorb vitamins A, D, E and K, so we cut it out of our diets at our peril.*

Okay-in-moderation foods

In this category, I would include a few items that are health-giving in some ways but whose disadvantages could easily outweigh the benefits if they are overindulged in. Also, some these items are best avoided in the early days if weight loss is still a priority. There are also a handful of items that aren't really Paleolithic in chronology but which, on balance, might not be too harmful if consumed sensibly. (This plan is about gaining benefits, not about recreating a historical period.)

Examples of these would be:

Chocolate – dark only, 70% cocoa or more. Avoid for weight loss but it does contain high levels of anti-oxidants to combat free radicals. Buy fair-trade if you're nice.

Red wine – Of all alcohols, red wine confers the most advantages. Like chocolate, it contains very high levels of anti-oxidants and, in moderation, is good for reducing stress. Consider two small glasses a day your limit though.

Tea and coffee – High levels of caffeine contribute to stress, high cortisone levels and skyward blood glucose levels; however, a cup or two of coffee or tea a day will do no harm. Non-organic coffee contains some of the highest levels of pesticide and herbicide of any household products, so always buy organic. Though classed as a stimulant, tea or coffee is always preferable to fizzy drinks, chemical-filled beers or grain-based spirits.

Honey – It turns out that eating local, raw, cloudy honey made from your local pollens may reduce hay fever symptoms by boosting your body's immunity (at least for as long as you remain in your region).[8] It's quite sugar-laden, so, even though it's natural sugar, you won't win any slimmer of the month awards if you feast on this year round. But as local honey is seasonal, you can't – see how clever nature is?

Healthy, heavier carbs – Foods are included under this heading because if you jump at these products before you have lost the weight you want to, you will not reach your ideal weight. Examples of healthy higher carbs that you can consume once your metabolism has recovered are **wild rice** (which is a grass, not a grain), **sweet potato**, **parsnips**, **quinoa** and **buckwheat** (which is technically a seed-based food).

You also might include some of these in your transition to a lower-carb eating plan as they can help avoid any temporary 'fug' or energy lag as your body switches to burning fat (and internal glucose), rather than the high-carb stuff it's accustomed to. People who keep excess weight off easily or those more interested in muscle gain than weight loss might include some of these items too. This sort of food is not essential for endurance events, however. No matter what conventional wisdom will tell you, "carb loading" is never required.

Dairy – This is a difficult one and a hotly disputed topic. Again it probably comes down to product quality and people's individual differences. Some people simply don't do well on milk, cheese and other dairy products. Many people find that when they cut these things out of their diet, long-standing conditions (like eczema, post-nasal drip or whatever else ails them) clear up within a week. Other people, however, seem to run on the stuff just fine.

Strictly speaking, Paleo is anti-dairy; however, I think the best policy is to cut dairy out of your diet for a month. Then, if all seems good, re-introduce it suddenly and heavily and note the effects. You might need to test cheese and milk separately. Like a good scientist, try not to change any other factors at the same time. If it seems to make no difference, then you're probably fine with dairy.

Having said that, there are still a few stipulations if you are going to enjoy milk and cheese: First, always go for **full-fat**. Semi-skimmed and skimmed milk is more heavily processed and is damaged in the heating process (rather like vegetable oil). It also doesn't contain the energy that you need to replace the heavy-carb you've now forsaken. Always choose **organic milk** or, if you can get it, drink **raw milk** (which is the holy nectar of milk). There is virtually no health risk with this if you get it from an established supplier. (Yes, it is legal. Search Google for your nearest farmer who makes deliveries). Raw milk is much richer in essential fats, protein, vitamins and minerals because it has avoided the pasteurization process that otherwise kills off most of its inherent goodness. Alternatively, **Guernsey and Jersey milk** (Gold Top) is superior to ordinary milk and is a good source of healthy fat if you don't mind the richer taste. Personally, I love it in coffee.

If you buy cheese, then look for **raw cheeses**, which are also unpasteurised and therefore keep their goodness.

A warning

Although I've just listed a number of tasty foods to be enjoyed in moderation, please don't forget that the bulk of your calories need to come from animal meat, fish, and eggs, along with plenty of vegetables. Only if you make this your focus will you end up with the health benefits and the body composition characteristics you are aiming for. Remember to get the basics right first. You are going to make a radical change in altering your main fuel from carbs to fat – a change your body will continue to thank you for the rest of your life, so don't compromise the benefits by looking for every easy indulgence you can find an excuse to consume before you've even got any steam up.

The other two elements of Instinctive Fitness (Natural Movement and Natural Lifestyle) are also massively important in the quest for fitness, health and happiness, but please remember: if the food you eat isn't right, then the other stuff will only get you so far. All three elements are supportive of each other and do not work nearly so well in isolation.

Key chapter points:

- *"Eat Naturally Edible Food" – organic/grass-fed meat, wild fish, eggs, local/organic vegetables, fruit, nuts, herbs and spices, and healthy oils.*

- *Don't eat grains, sugar, starches, margarines, vegetable oils, or industrially processed foods.*

- *Avoid all high-carb fare (even rice and sweet potato) until you've lost excess fat.*

- *Instead, get your energy from additional sources of fat, especially saturated fat (but avoid trans fats).*

- *Don't starve yourself to lose weight (it won't work in the long term). However, missing a meal and exercising instead once or twice a week will massively kick-start fat loss.*

- *Eat two or three times a day – no more.*

- *Buy the best quality, organic, free-range, local, grass-fed food you can afford.*

References:

1. Cuatrecasas P, Tell GPE (1973) "Insulin-Like Activity of Concanavalin A and Wheat Germ Agglutinin—Direct Interactions with Insulin Receptors." Department of Medicine, The John Hopkins University School of Medicine.

2. http://www.health-report.co.uk/saturated_fats_health_benefits.htm

3. Stender S, Dyerberg J (2004). "Influence of trans fatty acids on health". Ann. Nutr. Metab. 48 (2): 61–6. doi:10.1159/000075591. PMID 14679314.

4. Mozaffarian D, Rimm EB, Herrington DM. (2004) "Dietary fats, carbohydrate, and progression of coronary atherosclerosis in postmenopausal women." Am J Clin Nutr, 80(5): 1175-1184.

5. Eaton SB, Eaton SB 3rd, Sinclair AJ, Cordain L, Mann NJ (1998) "Dietary intake of long-chain polyunsaturated fatty acids during the Paleolithic Period." World Rev Nutr Diet, 12-23.

6. Machlin IJ, Bendich A, (1987) "Interesterification." FASEB Journal, 1:441-445 [Online] Available at: http://www. westonaprice.org/know-your-fats/556-interesterification.html; Enig, MG (1995) Trans Fatty Acids in the Food Supply: A Comprehensive Report Covering 60 Years of Research, 2nd Edition, Enig Associates, Inc, Silver Spring, MD, 148-154; Enig MG et al (1990) "Isomeric trans fatty acids in the U.S. diet." J Am Coll Nutr, 9(5):471-486.

7. The Weston A. Price Foundation (2012) "Soy Alert!" [Online] Available at: http://www.westonaprice.org/soy-alert. html.

8. Saarinen K, Jantunen J, Haahtela T. (2011) "Birch pollen honey for birch pollen allergy--a randomized controlled pilot study." Int Arch Allergy Immunol, 155(2):160-166.

CHAPTER ELEVEN

Natural Living

"If our nature is allowed to guide our life, we grow healthy, fruitful, and happy"
Abraham Maslow

In all the previous chapters we have looked mostly at what might be considered the 'hard' skills of Instinctive Fitness: the 'nitty-gritty' nuts and bolts of how to get your body into better shape.

This chapter is about taking a more rounded view: the 'soft' skills for a great life, if you like. Right back at the beginning of the book I claimed that Instinctive Fitness is not just another diet or exercise routine, and indeed it isn't. In this chapter I'd like to discuss how you could adopt a whole new lifestyle philosophy towards your own wellbeing and that of those around you.

This book has already suggested some new behaviours for getting your body in shape, but lifelong health involves more than just a good approach towards food and exercise. Feeling totally happy in yourself is perhaps only 50% about physical looks and performance, with the other half coming from having a relaxed outlook without undue stress.

> Our existence is nothing more than one big game: a game we're all going to ultimately lose sooner or later – so why not have a happy, playful, adventurous view on life while here?

Recap

Food is the easiest, most instantly effective improvement you can make to put the spring back in your step: change what you put in your mouth and change your whole life. What you consume is an area of your life you should be able to control with relative ease once you better understand those instincts that have previously been leading you astray. The food you choose to eat really can make an instant difference to how you look, feel and perform.

Try it and see.

Movement – we have already covered the hidden power of real movement at some length too; so this chapter attempts to outline other important factors that are not strictly about the body, but on which a truly happy, healthy life also depends.

Embracing a more natural existence

There are certain ways of living that are in harmony with our own nature as human animals. Where our lives deviate from the blueprint our genes expect, we set ourselves up to a greater or lesser extent for discomfort, disease and unhappiness.

Let's consider what sort of positive triggers our bodies expect to engage with. *Beyond proper nutrition and regular movement*, our genes expect a number of other things.

The following factors can be considered to be broadly **physical**:

- *Adequate rest and sleep*
- *Exposure to sunshine and outdoor life*

The following points are largely sociological or **psychological**; essentially they are strategies to combat the biggest life-wrecker and killer of all: long-term, uncontrolled **STRESS**:

- *Physical challenge and meaningful risk*
- *Play and festivity*
- *Other daily consumables (our chosen company, news, media, thoughts, etc)*
- *Love and belonging*

Stress: the silent killer

As discussed in earlier chapters, our 'fight or flight' stress response is totally natural and is there to give us a 'turbo boost' button when we need it most. Without a massively powerful reaction to moments of stress, ancient man would never have survived to pass on his genes to us.

During times of immediate danger from predators or during the excitement of the hunt they would have experienced what today would be called 'extreme stress': times when the 'fight or flight' mechanism is triggered. This response to stressful situations today enables us, just like our ancient ancestors, to reach new heights of performance – both physically and mentally. In times of high adrenalin the human body can perform at a higher level than normal and is capable of feats simply not possible in day-to-day life.

In a previous life my co-author was a fire-fighter and has experienced this adrenalin-fuelled 'high' many times. He once put the challenge to me to pick a fully-grown adult up from a seated position on the ground by lifting them under their arms with my hands. Not a chance, and nor can he normally. But in the line of duty, when the chips were down and with his body on high alert, he has done this many times without ever straining.

Stress and adrenalin are invaluable in short bursts when required, but *lethal* when inadvertently left switched on for months or even years.

Our cozy, modern world leaves us few opportunities to unleash our fight or flight instincts and crank our bodies up to the max. But our ancient bodies *yearn* to release these hormones from time to time to stay healthy. Today, with few dangers or 'chases' to perform, our stress response hormones 'leak' uncontrollably into our bloodstream.

It is accepted in modern medicine that stress is a key factor in many medical conditions and diseases. The ability to release these natural hormones in a controlled way through physical play and by indulging in intrinsically relaxing activities can reduce stress levels naturally without resorting to drugs.

Managing stress

For our hunter-gatherer ancestors, fitness, vitality and potency were not the intention of the lifestyles they lead; they were the by-products. Looked at 'instinctively', exercise is not a goal to be clawed for, simply time for physical play. A Paleo diet is not eaten just to make us look a certain way – but because it tastes better and makes us feel better than 'claggy', starch-filled products. Never mind the fact it's also far more nourishing.

> **Both eating and exercise should enjoyable activities you look forward to; if they are unpleasant or hurt – you're doing something wrong.**
> 'Instinctive' fitness is about daring to be more playful in your whole outlook on life; in the activities you participate in, in the food you cook and in the way you interact with other people.

World famous eastern/western medicinal health guru **Dr. Deepak Chopra** believes:

Prolonged stress can make you sick and can accelerate aging. Over time, the stress response can cause high blood pressure, heart disease, stomach ulcers, autoimmune diseases, cancer, anxiety, insomnia, and depression.

He goes even further with his assessment of conventional treatment for heart disease and says:

Since the early post-war era, many studies have found that being chronically stressed greatly increases your risk of heart disease, in part by raising circulating levels of cortisol, one of a number of "stress hormones." In fact, one study found that people with high levels of cortisol had five times the risk of dying from cardiovascular disease.
We believe that in having a more relaxed attitude toward the quest for health and fitness, and a playful attitude towards life as a whole, both mental and physical.[1]

On a long-term basis, thinking and fretting too much about exercise and nutrition can in itself be stressful and damaging. Anxiety and worry produce adrenaline in the body and that adrenaline has a corrosive long-term effect. Like a raucous, out of control party, it's exciting, exhilarating, and fun for an evening, but is not likely to do you, your health or your bank account a lot of favours if protracted over weeks or months.

The irony of this is that many of us seek the buzz of constantly high adrenaline levels, pursuing pseudo-high-octane activities like consoles games, movies, gambling or Internet surfing. Any of these activities in short bursts is arguably a good release of stress, but all too often the feel-good rush of adrenaline becomes an addiction in itself and can become all-consuming to the point of obsession. Adrenalin continuously pumping around the system is not good for the body and can result in an addiction to that activity.

> Any area of life where you just can't help yourself from over indulging, is one you should perhaps take a closer look at. Have your basic animal instincts been hijacked by modern hyper-stimuli beyond your control? Tread carefully.

The best tips for relaxation are to **slow down, do one thing at a time, and breathe evenly**. Relax your shoulder and neck muscles – if you can get your body to relax you'll soon find your mind follows. Too often we rush about, multi-tasking and worrying about stuff that usually never happens.

Staying present

For our ancestors, staying alive meant that they had no option but to stay tuned to the present moment to sense possible danger. This meant that they could not afford to indulge in any tendency towards daydreaming, introspection, over-analysis or worry. In doing so, they were able to appreciate what they had rather than dwelling on what they did not.

Many of the world's religions emphasise stillness, gratitude and awareness, usually through prayer and meditation. It seems to me that in doing so, they are fulfilling our deepest instinctive need for a greater experience of the present moment and a more profound reverence for life and nature. These practices fulfill a modern desire to escape from our endlessly churning, critical, verbally orientated mind, and to re-experience the sensation of observing life as it really happens.

Could it not actually be the calm, focused intensity and awareness of the hunter that is really missing in our lives?

An attitude of gratitude

Modern researchers into happiness and positive psychology repeatedly stress how important gratitude is in establishing a happy outlook. Without the influence of a consumer society, our historic predecessors would not have felt they wanted for much while there was a steady supply of food about. They thanked their Gods for favourable hunting outcomes and that increased their sense of gratitude and good fortune.

Today we are constantly bombarded with marketing messages from the media telling us what we're missing. It sells us stuff we don't need by making us feel that our lives are vitally lacking something. It makes us feel in some someway deficient and that we could instantly feel more worthy if we just whipped out the old credit card again.

It is my belief that a focus on **gratitude** and **life as it happens** is the beginning of the enlightened life. Our modern western mind is dominated by analytical thought, self-absorption and a lack of spontaneity. It's also plagued with rampant consumerism, with the message being that we can never have enough.

> "Work, work, work, buy, buy, buy" the media tell us. Without meaning to, we end up working harder than we want to, to buy stuff we don't need, for spare time we don't have, for a family we may rarely see.

Is it going too far to say that the hunter-gatherer ethos offers an alternative mental, emotional and spiritual model, as well as a superior physical one?

Adequate rest and sleep

In the quest for physical fitness, rest is often overlooked as a factor. Rest represents your body's chance to remake itself anew. Physical improvement is usually predicated on some sort of process of breakdown when the body is challenged and works overtime to repair and improve. If we train hard or work hard and do not allow adequate time for recovery, the result is overload and any gains are quickly reversed.

Ancient people left plenty of time for relaxing, having fun, playing and generally chilling out. They wouldn't have worked harder at the business of living than they absolutely had to – and yet today many people would look down upon this attitude; especially those whose identity is indelibly attached to their work. The self-denying, pleasure-denying, essentially Puritan character is still heavily engrained into our national psyche, making it very hard for us to just kick back, rest and enjoy ourselves.

There always seems to be something else that needs to be done before we can rest, assured of the fact that we are on the road to success. How many of us realize that chasing an abstract idea of "success" is like chasing the end of an ever-receding rainbow?

Sleep

Before the advent of timepieces, humans went to sleep when they felt tired, which was usually not long after nightfall. The cyclic nature of the day means that our natural hormonal balance shifts towards encouraging sleep after sunset. Most of us (despite modern trends) do not function well on fewer than eight hours sleep a day; short changing ourselves in this area has consequences much further reaching than short-term fatigue, we're also storing up multiple long-term health problems as well.

Most of the research on sleep points towards the idea that getting to bed early and rising with the sun is the most natural pattern to adopt. Interestingly, some research suggests that sleeping in two phases ('biphastically') might be the method most in line with our early history. This may have been an evolutionary adaptation that meant that there would always be someone awake (if only for an hour or two) during the night to watch out for the welfare of snoozing companions.

From this I take away the message that if I awaken during the night after going to sleep 'too early', I shouldn't worry about it, but should instead enjoy the peace and solitude before returning for the second portion of my night's R&R.

I like to keep my bedroom quite cool and my bed pretty warm; I think I sleep better this way. I don't set an alarm clock, but I wake up naturally soon after daybreak. If you've got things right you should wake up early, refreshed and ready to go.

If you went to bed early enough and stayed there long enough, but still found you didn't get a good eight hours of sleep, then it's time to experiment.

One thing to look at straight away is whether you spent your final hours awake staring at a TV or computer. If you did, the strength of the light will be telling your body that it's still the middle of day; so when you plunge it into the darkness of your bedroom it is far from prepared for sleep.

Gradually creeping darkness encourages the body to release hormones that slow the body down and relax the mind, in preparation for slumber. If you must watch TV, watch it in the early evening, rather than just before bed. If possible, gradually dim the lights through the evening with the use of dimmer switches or even candles on the dinner table. Or maybe – even more authentically – rely on the flickering light from a log fire in the hearth?

It's easy to gloss over the sleep issue: "Okay, so I don't sleep that well – so what?"

Poor sleep has a number of quite serious deleterious effects:

1. *It lowers our production of essential hormones like testosterone and growth hormone (which encourages the formation of adipose tissue through lower fat burning).*

2. *It maintains high stress levels (through higher levels of a hormone called cortisol) and therefore raises the risk of depression, high blood pressure and our susceptibility to diabetes and heart disease.*

3. *It reduces insulin sensitivity, meaning we handle the carbohydrates in our diet even worse, making it even harder to lose weight.*

When we sleep well, our immune system is strengthened, we lose fat, and physical and mental health improves.

So sleep well.

Exposure to sunlight and the outdoor life

In common with all creatures, humans were born to live outdoors. We have known for some time that people who rarely see sunlight (perhaps because they live inside the Arctic circle in winter or, more likely, because they have an office job) suffer from low levels of Vitamin D. UVB rays from the sun interact with cholesterol in our skin to produce what is actually an essential hormone affecting the functioning of our whole body.

Moreover, the right amount of sunlight is essential for building stronger bones and fighting osteoporosis, assisting fat loss, raising testosterone levels, strengthening the immune system, reducing inflammatory conditions and improving psychological wellbeing.

SAD (Seasonal Affective Disorder) has been well documented as a phenomenon affecting those who see little sunlight during the winter months. It has been hypothesised that this may account for the unusually high numbers of suicides in Scandinavia, even though these countries enjoy the highest standards of living in the world. Summer holidays do more than just offer rest and change; they also allow us to top-up our Vitamin D levels and shift our hormonal balance in a favourable direction.

Avoiding sunburn to lower the risk of skin cancer is essential, but hiding from sunlight entirely and only venturing outdoors occasionally – and then only slathered in Factor 40 sun block – makes no sense at all. Only by regularly getting large areas of skin exposed to moderate levels of UVB light can your body function at its best.

Recently, reports have begun to emerge that while protecting the skin, sun cream may actually be *damaging* children's health. Rickets, a disease that makes bones malleable and which was once thought to have been banished from this country, is increasingly popping up again on the healthcare radar. Caused again by a lack of Vitamin D, rickets was commonplace in the smog-shrouded, sun-deprived cities of the 19th century. Today, fearful parents won't let their children out of the house, or when they do they're smothered from head to foot in factor 50, which reflects much of the sun's vitamin forming rays.

Long before we shackled ourselves to the clock and the 'working day', ancient humans would surely have behaved like all the other animals: rising early with sun, doing their day's hunting and gathering when the day was cool, and taking shelter as the sun climbed in the sky to avoid dehydration and sunburn. They wouldn't have had the need of the farmer to toil all day in the fields, but instead would have enjoyed a shorter working day surrounded by nature's bountiful larder.

Without sun cream, the *fear* of sunshine or the *pressure* to wear sun cream, they would surely have enjoyed a deep year-round tan, built up slowly and carefully over a lifetime.

In terms of the outdoor life, humans developed in various different environments, but all of them were natural rather than man-made. We are more relaxed and in-touch with ourselves in natural surroundings. Physical contact with nature and animals gives us a sense of reconnecting with something that is painfully missing in the artificial banality of urban life.

Take home message: you need nature and sunshine to thrive. Get away from urban life and enjoy sunshine sensibly in a natural environment whenever possible.

Physical challenge and meaningful risk

In a world increasingly obsessed with ''elf and safety', finding anything remotely risky to do when getting physical is not an easy task. When we were young (especially us boys) we liked to lay it all on the line when the opportunity arose: climbing a tall tree, venturing into a field with a bull, playing games we really shouldn't in derelict buildings – all just for the thrill.

Today, as adults, we've had "Is it safe?' hammered into us to the extent that our natural instinct to take a calculated risk for worthwhile reward has been all but squashed. We now get our 'kicks' cheaply and second-hand from films, television and video games.

All these imposters are designed to fire up the 'fight or flight' adrenalin kick we all so enjoy, and are our sterile and safe modern world's way of offering a cheap thrill without ever actually laying safety on the line. We all yearn to be scared from time to time – why else would film studios rake in huge profits producing films that are frankly designed to do nothing else but scare the pants off us?

It should come as no surprise that the stars of sports such as Formula One, Moto GP and boxing are some of the best paid and most revered. Take the driver out of a racing car and control it remotely from the pits and it simply doesn't have the same allure. We love it that our hero's prepared to pay the ultimate price for the glory, because at heart we ourselves would die for the same thrill.

NASA never strictly *needed* to send a man to the moon to achieve its scientific objectives. But NASA did need to pay for all the fun and games it was planning. To do that, it needed money – and lots of it. The only way to persuade the taxpayers of America to stump up the *billions* of dollars required to get them into space was to sell the general public a dream; so they captured their imagination by offering up modern day gladiators – heroes prepared to risk it all on top of a 111 meter high, 129 tonne 15,700 mph bomb.

Instinctive Fitness isn't about being shot at the moon or even climbing up the outside of a tower block without a rope; it's not about taking foolish risks just for a kick, but it is about stretching your mental and physical limits.

Fun risk and reward activities – not exercise

Any physical activity undertaken with the true spirit of Instinctive Fitness involves not only some sort of movement but a challenge: an element of risk and reward that is controlled and exciting rather than laborious or dangerous.

- *How about the 'rush' of sprinting down a steep hill faster than you feel comfortable with, risking a tumble?*

- *How about pull-ups hanging from a footbridge above a small stream – no danger but the very real risk of getting cold and wet.*

- *What about a game of paintball with a sizable forfeit. Imagine the intensity of the experience when the consequences of being hit are cleaning the victor's car inside and out.*

What other risk and reward games can you think of? Please let us know your ideas at info@instinctive-fitness.com

Instinctive training should, wherever possible, have an element of risk, reward and exhilaration, although in reality no real danger. Any form of exercise should leave you feeling better than before you started. Not just because it's a better way of gaining any fitness goals you may have, but because we want our brain to keep dragging us back – associating exercise with pleasure not pain.

There are many other activities that are great for enjoying in themselves and provide fantastic fitness benefits. Obviously, unless you're very rich and have plenty of 'play time', some of these are unlikely to form part of your daily activities but, should you get the chance, they fall right into the Instinctive Fitness ethos.

* tree climbing * skateboarding * paintballing * mountain biking * wild swimming * go-cart racing * bouldering * martial arts * 'capture the flag' * rock jumping * friendly wrestling * free-running * surfing * white water canoeing * paddle boarding * teasing crocodiles *

Just kidding with the last one – but you get the point.

The fight or flight experience

Obviously it's not wise to replicate the conditions that set off a true fight or flight mechanism just for training's sake. However, by playing a psychological game, 'fight or flight' training actually replicates the exhilaration and heightened physical response called for in times of crisis.

We believe that allowing the body to run at its real maximum capacity for just a minute or two at a time provides a host of health benefits over the long term. Giving the adrenal gland the chance to switch into full flow and giving the body a chance to operate at flat-out maximum pace enables the adrenalin to shut off completely when we don't need it, allowing the body to relax properly afterwards.

Check out www.instinctive-fitness.com for more ideas on great ways to have fun while unintentionally getting fit.

Play and festivity

Although hunter-gatherers endured some tough times, these were matched by plenty of time for play, fun and relaxation. The natural way to celebrate a big kill was with a big feast. When they overcame genuine challenges (rather than the artificial type we know today, like 'surviving' an internal audit), their relief was easily expressed in dancing, joy, festivity and rest.

Today, many of us struggle to exert ourselves, even once a week – and yet find it harder still to truly relax when we want to. Tension and a feeling of dissatisfaction are almost endemic in our world where we are neither fully physically challenged nor truly at rest. We need this 'Yin and Yang' to enable us both to 'switch on' fully and to 'switch off' fully. This middle ground malaise is quite simply sabotaging our time to recharge, lose our self-consciousness and truly celebrate just being.

Our lives are becoming increasingly regimented, ordered, measured and made to march to a timetable. Try adding more opportunities for just messing about, exploring, having fun, and generally just being playful. Climb a tree, put on a play with your kids, write a poem, chase your dog in circles – it doesn't matter much.

Spontaneous playfulness is at the heart of creativity; it's the spark of genius at the centre of both our social and working lives – if only we could just stop being so uptight about productivity and tap its creative energy.

Living a natural life isn't just in the details – it's in the spirit. Loosen up a bit. Get out and do things; experience things. Spend less time worrying about being able to afford stuff. What you can't afford is to miss this precious time you have alive. Relax and enjoy what you have. Appreciate the good things and the good people you already have in your life.

Other consumables

Food and drink are not the only things we input into the body; we also consume other people's ideas, attitudes and versions of truth.

Other influences that dictate our health, our fitness and our very being include:

- *the company we keep*

- *the TV we watch*

- *the papers delivered*

- *the books we read*

- *the music we listen to*

- *even the thoughts we think*

Our little blue spinning planet has lots of stuff going on – some good things and some bad things – but ultimately, it's only the things you pay attention to which make up *your* unique experience of the world.

The information you ingest forms your opinion on what the world is all about.

When fear, resentment, aggression and other negative influences fill up your consciousness – your whole perception of the world *becomes* fear, resentment and aggression.

When you surround yourself with contentment, generosity and harmony, your life becomes contentment, generosity and harmony.

Which do *you* want?

Hanging out with negative people, watching tragedy-filled soap operas, reading horror and murder novels, listening to angst-filled music, will all eventually make up the foundations of the thoughts you think and the feelings you feel.

Why would anyone *want* to watch a modern, British soap opera? Why on earth does a large percentage of Britain's population choose to have their evenings filled with tragedy, rivalry and back-biting? And why do so many people watch the eternal doom and gloom of the 10 O'clock news before they go to bed? No matter which channel you watch, all news programs gloss over all the good things – the successes, the triumphs, the lives saved and the philanthropy – because it doesn't win viewing figures.

The media makes money pumping a relentless supply of caustic news and drama into our front room – and we passively take the bait.

The point of this very small section of the book is not to pass judgment on what's good, bad, right or wrong or what you should and should not pay attention to – but simply to draw your attention to where your attention is being drawn.

Like the food you put into your body, please think carefully about the messages you put into your mind, as it is these that ultimately influence and shape your whole life. Choose carefully what you watch, be discerning as to what you listen to, and carefully consider those people whose opinions you allow to influence your own.

Love (and loyalty and support)

At the risk of sounding a bit soppy, I'll remind you that Abraham Maslow (possibly the best known positive psychologist of all time) considered all the forms of love to be one of the central tenets in his famous hierarchy of human needs. (By now you'll have noticed that I love anything in a pyramid!)

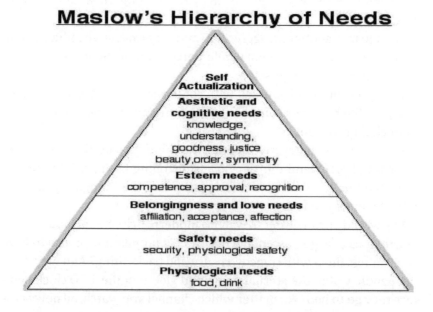

In a very real sense we can say that every human needs love. (The Beatles, of course, were right when they sang: "All you need is love") Going back thousands of years, every human could expect love, cherishing, and validation; a sense of identity provided by their tribe, family and chosen partner. They lived in an era when each and every day they could prove their worth, and from their actions they knew their place in the order of things. They understood directly what they brought to the table and what they brought to the world.

For our ancestors, to be without any sort of love was to die; to be cast out of the tribe and wander until dead. Nowadays our fate may not be sealed in the same way, but a need to be cherished, approved of and appreciated never leaves us, no matter how grown up we might think ourselves. A life without love is one without meaning or direction. It descends to a basic level of fulfilling desires, characterised by shallow, selfish thinking and growing disillusion.

These days, we suffer from a fractured sense of tribal loyalty. We are still expected to show loyalty to our families, but also now to our employers, our nation, our chosen shopping brands, our political parties, our sports teams and our unique British sense of class. With so many different pulls on our affection, it's very hard these days to know what we really do stand for. A true sense of belonging is increasingly rare. However, it is, was and always will be a very special thing indeed for anybody who finds it.

If you feel I am getting off-point with this thread, it's worth pointing out that since we appeared on this little planet pretty much the one subject that there is a consensus on from all purveyors of wisdom is that positive, balanced emotions are the backbone of good health; and that corrosive stressful emotions, such as loneliness, anger and sadness, are linked to weaker immune systems and a higher chance of developing serious illnesses.

Life is short and offers us but a small window of opportunity to feast on all its glories. Don't spend the years you do have worrying, stressing and feeling fearful. Seize the day! Every day, think and do nurturing things – and the rewards of health, fitness and happiness will offer themselves willingly.

Key chapter points:

- *Sleep well – it matters. Get your eight hours or whatever your body needs. Get your body-clock back in line with the sun.*

- *Take time to relax in the evenings and at moments through the day.*

- *Get more sunshine (but don't get burnt)*

- *Take on sensible physical challenges and meet them with awareness and present-moment focus.*

- *Stop stressing about things in the future, which will never happen.*

- *Include time for fun, celebration and playfulness. There should be a time to have fun and be silly – it's a serious matter. Try exercising in a playful manner.*

References

1.http://www.deepakchopra.com/blog/view/52/heart_attack_myths_and_the_missing_x_factor_

CHAPTER TWELVE

Putting it all together

"Knowing is not enough, we must apply. Willing is not enough, we must do".
Bruce Lee

Just to recap, there are three main areas that you should look at if you intend to completely overhaul your physical condition:

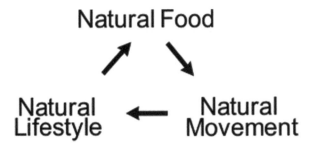

We will look at each one in turn and show how you can gain the most benefits from each with the least expenditure of effort. To use an ugly American phrase, how to get the most 'bang for your buck'. What this chapter will do is lay down a path that will be suitable for most people, most of the time. If you are an international rugby star or have difficulties walking, then these approaches may not be optimal, but the principles will still hold true.

Change your exercise: natural movement

Let's have another look at the Instinctive Fitness exercise pyramid where the activities at the base represent the activities you should pursue most frequently; and those at the uppermost tip, the least.

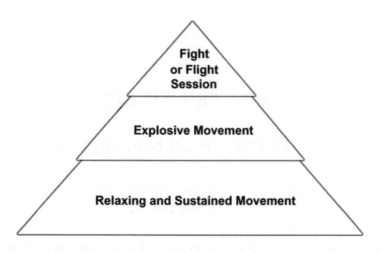

Outlined in the pyramid are suggested times you should aim for: what I call the minimum effective dose. Some people who really want to put in the effort could do a lot more than this and still only get 20-25% fitter. The law of diminishing marginal returns kicks in quite quickly, so 'more' is optional depending on your lifestyle, goals and temperament.

You might like to make your week's activities look something like this:

Monday: *Explosive Movement* or heavy resistance task (12-25 minutes)
Tuesday: *Relaxed, Sustained* walk (40 minutes+) or rest if tired
Wednesday: *Fight or Flight* session (15 minutes, before or instead of low-carb breakfast)
Thursday: *Relaxed, Sustained* game of tennis, nine holes of golf or walk (40 minutes+) or rest if tired
Friday: *Explosive Movement* or heavy resistance task or strong resistance task (12-25 minutes)
Saturday: *Relaxed, Sustained* five mile country/park walk (2 hours), or round of golf
Sunday: Rest/play

This might look, at a glance, like an ordinary programme, but it's not. What's special about the above – and alternatives based around the same pyramid – is:

- *This programme doesn't have the one-sided bias towards any one single quality that most do. It's a programme for* **total all-round development***. It's got all three of the different movement intensities we looked at in the Natural Movement chapter.*

224

- *The movements are all natural without any muscle groups being isolated.*

- *The quantities and proportions are right – you won't burn out or fail to challenge yourself.*

- *There's plenty of recovery built in (3 days a week of rest if you need it).*

- *It's totally adaptable for what you like to do, your energy levels and your mood. The 'golf' and 'tennis' mentioned above were just examples. Just exchange them for activities of a roughly equal intensity that you personally enjoy.*

- *It's enjoyable because it's customizable. You'll want to come back and do it again – as well as try new things if your interests wane.*

Posture and good alignment

As we have previously discussed, posture and flexibility are the foundations upon which all the other areas of IF exercise are built. The type of exercise that Instinctive Fitness encourages in itself promotes good posture and flexibility. However let's run through a few areas you might like to look at to get you started.

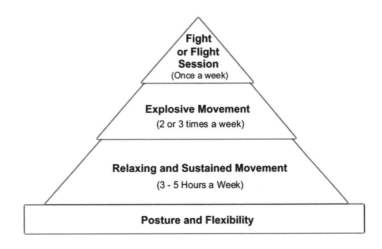

Posture is something that needs to be worked on constantly, but it doesn't actually require any specific time at all – just constant vigilance and awareness. You will need some help with this though – at least initially, until you are practising the right way. To get onto the right lines, I advise you to purchase the book by Esther Gokhale called **8 Steps to a Pain-Free Back**. Esther's principles, instructions and pictures will soon have you on the way to a better posture and all-round improved performance. It is required reading for everyone from grandmothers to international athletes.

Buy it even if your back doesn't hurt now – if you follow her eight steps it will change your life forever.

Lie, walk, sit and stand – naturally

Following Esther's principles, built up over years of studying the postures of nations and cultures with no incidence of postural difficulties, is the single best thing you can do to guard against the ravages of old-age and spinal atrophy. I can't recommend it highly enough. If you're reading this in the UK, there are now teachers of her method here as well as in the USA.

Even if you don't buy the book, there's still plenty you can do to help yourself out:

- *Don't spend hours slumping in chairs*
- *Stand to work if you can (I am standing as I write this)*
- *Get up frequently to stretch and move about*
- *Take mini-breaks to get fresh air or march up and down the office stairs every 40 minutes or so*
- *Explore simple stretches, movements and mini-workouts you can do throughout the day in five-minute chunks*

Almost any movement will stop your discs totally compressing in the way they certainly will when sitting with your body in poor alignment; some exercises and stretches are much more effective than others though.

Two simple things you can do to improve your posture right now are to remember not to push your hips forward when you stand or to allow your tailbone to tuck under when you sit. Even in a seated position, your bottom should retain its distinctive 'bottom-like' shape. If it disappears when you sit down, you're not doing yourself any postural favours.

Another idea – shoot me if you think this is terribly old-fashioned – is to place a beanbag on your head and balance it there while you go about your day. This is what African ladies have learned to do to maintain their exemplary posture, except that they tend to do it with enormous jars of water rather than with beanbags. Now don't get me wrong, I'm not suggesting you do this in the office or in public – you'll get funny looks – but in the privacy of your own home this little tip works pretty well. It stops you poking your head forward so much and pushing your hips in front. It also encourages better balance by encouraging you to glide rather than bounce up and down when you move.

As you become more aware of how you move around, try to get into the habit of hip-hinging when you bend for things. Learn to bend at the hips rather than in the back to pick things up. Don't bend your knees much unless you have to reach very low. Instead your hips should move backwards from their position over your feet in order for your upper body to become more horizontal.

Check out our website at www.instinctive-fitness.com; it's always being updated with new information on this sort of thing.

Sq-what?

The other essential movement that you need to work into your day more is the squat. This is a movement that our ancestors would have performed many times a day (especially when sitting around a fire). Include it in your workouts or use it in your mini-work breaks. Work up to the full squat by putting a two inch raised block under the heel of each foot. Mix them up by doing ordinary ones, wide ones, narrow ones, ones with your left foot forward, right foot forward and every combination in between. Then do it on uneven ground. You get the idea: variety is the key here. The increased strength and flexibility this will bring your legs and hips is extraordinary.

Walking

> "Walking is the best exercise. Habituate yourself to walk very far"
> **Thomas Jefferson**

Walking gives us many of the same benefits as traditional aerobic activity (calorie burning, lowered blood pressure, lowered resting heart rate, increased cardiac output, increased capillary density, increased nutrient/oxygen delivery, etc.) without all of the drawbacks (musculoskeletal injury, joint wear and tear, elevated stress hormones, muscle loss, lowered metabolic rate, etc.). Simply put, it's the aerobic activity we were born to do.

If you're going to be doing plenty of this then it makes sense to do it well. That means doing it as we evolved to. There could be a whole book on this subject, but a few basic principles will get you up and, er, walking.

First footwear: minimalist type shoes are best to keep you in touch with the ground and your feet working as they should. You will find a range of recommended shoes on the Instinctive Fitness website. Even if you decide these aren't for you, ensure that your footwear has a thin, soft-ish, flat sole with plenty of room for your toes to spread. Avoid heavy shoes with any sort of elevated heel. A simple pair of old-school gym shoes is still better for your health, poise and co-ordination than the best pair of Nikes. Just because you can't feel the impact of the road much in high-end trainers doesn't mean it's not there.

However, damage to your joints will accrue more slowly wearing cushioned shoes than if you carelessly slam your heels down in just the same way in paper-thin soles, so it's important that, as in days of yore, when stalking was a skill and not a criminal offence, you learn to tread softly and quietly again.

To encourage a natural stride, ensure that one foot is placed roughly in-line with the next, as if you were walking along a single white line. Having feet that run on two different tracks means that you lack balance and flexibility in your hips. Make sure you don't hold tension in your legs as you walk. If your head wobbles from side to side as you walk, or bounces up and down more than half-an-inch, you need to work on your technique and posture.

When you are walking well, you should feel your bum muscles contract as you take each step, rather than feeling the need to lift each foot and place it in front of you. Good walking should feel like it happens almost by itself.

Running

Good technique is hard to get a grip on until you can walk well, but up-right balance is the key. Most of us hunker forward when we run, lead-ing with our heads and tucking our pelvis under as we move. We tend to focus on pushing off with each long-stride rather than taking shorter-strides, cushioned by a little controlled bend in the knees.

If you really want to master this and run with the easy languid gait of a Kenyan miler or the effortless grace of Usain Bolt, I suggest you seek out a "Pose" running specialist near you. However if you work on your basic posture throughout the day, there will be some good transference to all your movements, including running technique.

The most essential principle is that your feet should be placed under-neath you when running, not in front. Most people throw their feet out in front of themselves and then tumble forward on to them. They typically bounce up and down as they run and often sway from side to side too. This is wrong and is caused mainly by the harmful modern habit of heel-striking, which is only made possible by modern running shoes. (Yet another example of how modern technology has hindered more than helped)

Heel-striking (landing on the heel and rolling forwards in each step) has only been possible since the advent of the cushioned running shoe 40 years ago and represents the single biggest cause of running injuries. Heels striking the ground in cushioned shoes (80% of runners) impact with three times the force of those habituated to barefoot running.[1] Is it any wonder that there are so many injuries these days?

A minimalist shoe is a good compromise, but slapping your heels down in a shoe that has no cushioning is a very quick way to injury. You need to get your form right, relearning how to run on the balls of the feet with your body upright and your feet circling beneath you. Your heels should only touch down lightly, after the balls of your feet have made contact with the ground, before being pulled up quickly underneath your hips again.

One of the quickest ways to improve running technique is to practise occasionally without any shoes at all. (This is the way you were born to run.) A slightly rough surface underfoot will soon have you cushioning every landing with the natural bend of your knees and the flexibility in the arch of your forefoot.

Having said that, if you transition to a minimalist shoe (or bare footing) too fast, and don't allow time for your softer forefoot-strike to catch up, you could end up injuring yourself. Be careful and get advice before embarking.

For more information on 'barefooting', see the work of Daniel Lieberman, Professor of Human Evolutionary Biology at Harvard University.[1]

Change your eating style: eat natural food

For improving your body shape and staying free from illness, changing the way you eat is more powerful than any other single change you can make.

Here's how you could do it:

1. Clear your cupboards

A natural food fascist would have you go through all the food in the house and chuck out everything that doesn't have a place in the following food triangle. But we're going to be more pragmatic than that and you'll get a whole week to get your kitchen in order:

Putting the right food into your kitchen and getting rid of the stuff you don't want to be eating is half the battle.

This means you will over the coming week either use up or chuck out:

All processed-foods, vegetable oils (and products containing them), grains (cereals, breads, biscuits, pasta, etc.), starches (including potatoes), sugars, margarines, table salt, skimmed and semi-skimmed milk, pasteurised cheeses, beans, mayonnaise, jams, spreads, malt drinks, fizzy drinks, energy drinks [*takes deep breath*] and concentrated fruit juices.

You will want a kitchen that contains at least an oven, a hob, a kettle, a microwave and maybe a grill and slow-cooker. You can eBay the toaster by the way; you won't need it anymore.

2. Put clean, fresh foods into your kitchen

The next step is to go and hit the shops, but with a new state of awareness. Alternatively you can get great food delivered. However, if you want the very best, it's frankly not much use heading to the supermarket. Specialist farmers will deliver a higher standard of meat and veg (organic as well as grass-fed). If all this five-star dining is outside your financial reach, then you will do okay at Tesco, Waitrose, Sainsbury's or any of the other big supermarkets, but you will need to move through them like a racehorse wearing blinders, shopping wisely.

Here's a visual remind of what you're looking for:

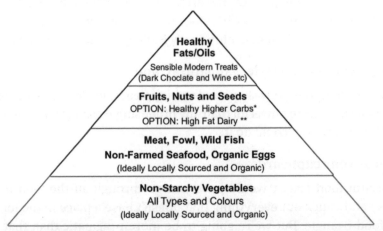

* e.g. sweet potato, wild rice, buckwheat – good, if not looking to lose weight
** Be sure to do a withdrawal test to ensure dairy works with your digestive system

Remember: the pyramid is arranged by recommended food *volume*, not calories. You should eat more of those foods at the 'base' of the pyramid than those at the top.

If you are using a supermarket you'll find that most of the aisles contain foods which, according to my definition, are just 'bait' foods – i.e. they look appealing, but actually aren't fully edible (because nature didn't provide them for our consumption). Luckily, supermarkets tend to put these products in the middle of the shop. Most of what you will want is concentrated around the periphery of the building.

You will want to hit the grocery section really hard for fruit and vegetables (don't stray into the bread section) before making for the fresh or frozen meat section. When buying meat, look for a variety of different animal types (including fowl and game). Choose big joints, large racks of ribs, or other large portions. Buying in bulk like this will keep down both costs and time spent preparing foods, as I'll explain shortly. Always choose organic if you can afford it. (It's worth it, so consider your priorities)

After that, you will want to choose some fresh or frozen fish, some frozen vegetables or berries (for convenience) and possibly pick up a few bottles of organic, whole-fat milk.

Next you'll need to find some 'healthy' fat for cooking. Look for lard, goose fat, butter (organic), coconut oil, ghee (hard to find) or other animal fat. Additionally, choose a high-quality extra virgin olive oil for salads.

If you need any flour for bulking up dishes, choose coconut flour, almond flour, or ground arrowroot (these are all unprocessed, ground products).

You'll also want to pick up some eggs and some bacon. High-end burgers and sausages can now also be found that are 100% beef and free from gluten (breadcrumbs), so these are okay too.

When you get home, you will find that these will mostly, being fresh products, need to go into the fridge or freezer. Freeze all of the meat apart from some bacon and whatever meat you will cook next. The more freezer space you have here the better. Only a few things, like herbs, will need cupboard space.

3. Plan ahead for every meal

Evening meal (you'll see why I'm listing this first in a moment)

Choose a meal the whole family will enjoy. Take time to consider making something special. This is the most important meal; it's ideal if everyone is present and sits around the table. (If you don't social-ise at meal times, when will you?) You should have defrosted your chosen meat (or fish) prior to the time you start to put the meal together.

Take time to check out a recipe book or just have fun improvising if you're a creative or carefree cook. Don't forget that your meal will need to be composed of about two thirds vegetables and one third meat/fish/eggs. (In terms of calories it's more like 40/60 though).

I'll suggest some meal options in a minute, but the important thing is to cook loads of meat, certainly more than your family can possibly eat at one sitting, and place it on a large platter in the middle of the table. Then let people help themselves to the meat and the veg, taking as much or as little as they want. It may be a bit of a culture shock if you're used to bringing portioned plates to the table, but here are the advantages:

- *Everyone has the chance to eat until they are full.*

- *No one leaves the table hungry.*

- *Nobody ends up eating more than they feel like just because the family custom is that all the food is finished.*

- *There is plenty of meat left over for at least a meal or two the next day, which means you save on cooking time. Simply jazz it up a bit and re-serve.*

- *It justifies buying large joints, which means you can buy meat more economically.*

We all do this 'cheat' at Christmas, so why not the rest of the year?

If you want to save even more kitchen time, buy a slow cooker. At lunchtime, get someone to chop up some vegetables and throw them into the pot, add lots of meat. Then leave it for 4-9 hours. The beauty of this is that food is ready to eat whenever you want it. You can then eat immediately when you get home in the evening if you wish. You don't have to be present while it cooks.

Another advantage of this is that if you can't all be present for sup-per (shame on you), family members can serve themselves whenever it suits them.

232

Breakfast

This tends to be the meal most people struggle with because we are all so accustomed to reaching for a quick bowl of cereal, toast or croissant. Please, whatever you do, avoid carbs here. Instead, look to make something with eggs, fruit, fish, or light meats (an idea that Europeans find easy).

You could even have a 'Traditional English' minus the toast and hash browns. Tuck into eggs, either scrambled or fried in butter or lard; add some bacon, grilled mushrooms, grilled tomato, quality sausages, chicken liver – whatever you fancy. Perhaps you could have a plain omelette or something with tuna, or a simple fruit salad – or just dig back into some meat from last night's supper. With just a few extra minutes and a little bit of imagination you really can set your day off to a great start.

Lunch

This is your opportunity to get loads of flavor-full and nutrient-loaded vegetables inside you. It's also a chance to ensure you get a good supply of satiating protein and fat into your stomach. I recommend that you make a massive salad. Cut up every vegetable in sight and throw them into a salad bowl, then add some meat from last night's feast. Or you could fry up some fish quickly. Throw in a few nuts, seeds and some grapes. Add a dressing made of virgin olive oil, lemon juice and sea salt; add any other spices that take your fancy. If you don't eat it all, you can refrigerate it and use it as a side-salad for your evening meal.

At this point I'm often asked *"What actual meals can I eat? Are there any meals that will excite me? I mean, what does that leave?"*

Here's my non-exhaustive list as a response to that. Most of these might be considered 'suppers' (or 'dinners'), but they could just as easily be eaten for lunch as well if you have the time to prepare them.

Meal options and ideas

(Just add more veg)

Hotpot (Chicken/lamb/pork)	*Garlic lamb kebabs (on a stick) with veg*
Curry with cauliflower rice	*Baked fish*
Beef stir-fry	*Grilled chops/fish/steak*
Roast chicken/beef/pork with	*English breakfast – bacon, sausage, onion,*
Roast vegetables	*mushroom, tomato*

BBQ chicken and salad

Steamed halibut and veg

Beef burgers (100% beef) with mixed frozen veg

Meatballs and sautéed fresh tomatoes

Chilli-con-carne with tomato

Pork and apple casserole

Lamb tagine

Grilled beef heart with roasted peppers

Curried salmon salad

Slow cooked pork-stuffed peppers

Omelette with bacon

Prawn salad

Rabbit and onion casserole

Salt and pepper squid

Aromatic whole grilled chicken

Sesame chicken and "rice"

Shrimp, sausage and summer squash casserole

Cajun style blackened chicken liver and lemon and garlic sauce

Thai green curry

Lobster, grapefruit and avocado salad

Scrambled egg and smoked salmon

Sausage casserole

Bacon, chicken and avocado salad

Tender beef tongue with onion and garlic

Bacon, egg, tomato and avocado salad

Pork tenderloin with cilantro pesto

Medallions of lamb with spinach

Beef goulash

Garlic-pulled pork

Zesty lemon-and-lime seafood salad

Sushi

Stir-fry liver with courgettes

Frittata aleta

Arctic chowder

Organic prawn curry

Chicken and shrimp soup

Watercress and bacon soup

Beef stroganoff with deep-fried cauliflower

Grilled spareribs with boiled asparagus

Oxtail casserole with Brussels sprouts

Peppered salmon steaks

Stuffed marrow/butternut/tomatoes/onion/squash – best with mince

Kippers with avocado puree

Tuna salad with broccoli

Italian spinach flan with Brussels sprouts

Steamed scampi

Mushroom stuffed with lamb's kidney

Pork escalope

Salmon steak in red wine

Kidneys in sherry sauce with stuffed peppers

Oriental stir-fry with coconut sauce

Tiger prawn curry and cauliflower rice

Lobster/crab

BBQ'd pork and green pepper brochettes

Lamb offal with pureed carrots

Baked herring

Sausages, grilled, with mixed vegetables, steamed

Lamb casserole

Summerset style pork

Prawn and pear salad

Chilli pork with leeks in red wine

Thai stir-fried vegetables with meat of choice

Curried aubergines

Foil-baked bas

Lamb ratatouille	*Chicken a la king*
Tossed green salad with avocado	*Haddock/cod/salmon – instantly cook-*
Red cabbage campagnard with bacon-	*able in microwave with veg of choice*
Sauerkraut	*Greek vegetable soup*
Liver pâté	

For more recipe ideas, please visit www.instinctive-fitness.com/recipes

Free your palette

If you don't find much in the list that whets your appetite, then you're probably still addicted to the carbohydrates prevalent in your current diet. Given time, you will come to notice the 'claggy', heavy texture of bread and other grain-based products, and you'll regain your instinct and taste for real food.

When transitioning to low-carb, it is possible to go too far, too soon. If you do, you will start to feel a low-energy 'fug' and possibly suffer from grotty moods. Don't worry, it is only temporary and will probably only last a few weeks. You can make the transition easier by allowing yourself some healthy carbs, such as wild rice, sweet potato, or quinoa, when you need them. However, if you overdo the carbs you'll not lose any weight at all, so please be judicious. Ensuring you include more fat in your diet and not just extra protein is essential if you are going to have a chance of feeling normal during the transition phases. If in doubt, two or three table spoons of coconut oil a day will fire up your new fat burning metabolism nicely.

Obviously you also need to be careful in how you prepare these foods. You need to make these meals entirely at home (no microwave versions out of tin trays) and you mustn't add banned ingredients. Try not to add corn flour to your dishes, for instance; instead use the alternative bulking ingredients already mentioned. Most of these meals are delicious, simple to make and have recipes freely available on the Internet by Googling "Paleo recipes". Any recipes that are part of the Paleo health movement will be suitable for you. There are many on Marks Sisson's superlative website www.marksdailyapple.com. There are also lots more inspirational pictures of personal transformations based on this way of eating than I can possibly fit in this book.

If you're still not sure that you're eating the right way or you're worried you're not getting the weight loss you want as fast as you would like

(1-2 pounds a week is great progress, by the way), then there is a pain-less way to check you're on the right track.

Open an account with a website like www.fitday.com. Input all your details and, for two or three representative days, record every morsel of food that you eat after each meal. This isn't as hard as it may sound – drop down menus make it very easy. With this tool you will be able to see how much carbohydrate you're really ingesting.

You'll probably need to get this well below 200g a day for success. Somewhere near 150 grams is usually right. If you drop much lower than this, this would indicate that you are not actually eating enough vegetables because, remember, these are still carbohydrates – just not densely packed ones.

Use a system like this to ensure you've got things about right and then, pretty quickly, you will develop a feeling for what works for you and what doesn't. At that point you can give up the task of data entry after each meal.

Although Paleo-style eating may sound like a shock to the system, and perhaps, for those used to instant food, a bit of a faff to prepare, it really isn't. With just a bit of strategic preparation and a new philosophy behind it, this way of eating is easily worth the minor effort involved.

Four Sample Days of Living 'Instinctively'

Below you'll find the outline of a few days in your life should you chose to live 'instinctively'. It's not intended as a prescription, just a flavour of how food and exercise can be worked into the average week.

MONDAY:

Wake ½ hour earlier than you do currently and get the day started with a glass of filtered water followed by **25 minutes of Explosive Movement training**.

Breakfast: You boil six eggs, eating 3 soft boiled immediately with some butter, spinach and salt and pepper to taste; the others are left to hard boil and are saved for lunch. *You indulge in a cup organic coffee to wash it all down. A mini-work break mid-morning sees you knocking out one or two of a variety of different kinds of squats without working up a sweat. You drink another pint of water before 10am.*

Lunch: You eat the 3 put-aside, hard-boiled eggs with a tuna salad, including mushrooms, onions, peppers, cucumber, broccoli, grapes, and plenty of greens with some olive oil and balsamic vinegar. *After lunch you go for a 10 minute brisk walk outdoors while leisurely drinking a pint of water over the afternoon. Being slightly peckish later, you eat a handful of macadamia nuts.*

Supper: Comprises as much of a large roast chicken or joint of beef (with masses of steamed and buttered cauliflower, courgette and carrot) as you fancy. You switch the *TV or computer off soon after eight pm, relax and read with the lights lowered for the rest of the evening. You head to bed when feeling sleepy and are asleep by 9.45pm.*

TUESDAY:

You rise early for a Relaxed, Sustained walk (30 to 40 minutes).

Breakfast: Fruit-salad.

Lunch: Chicken (or beef) salad with last night's leftovers, using lots of romaine lettuce, cherry tomatoes, radishes, onion, bell peppers, avocado and various green vegetables. (Score extra points if you include avocado and the excellent fats it contains). If you get hungry in the afternoon, you try bottled olives as a snack, or have some more macadamia nuts. (You don't eat these if you're not hungry though).

Supper: None – just skip it and go to bed a little earlier. If you're new to this way of eating you might hold off on this little fast until the rest of the programme is second nature. *Other details the same as in the italics above.*

WEDNESDAY:

You enjoy an eight minute Fight or Flight session (using Tabata protocol – plus five minute warm-up and five minute warm down) on bicycle or on foot. You would consider doing this barefoot if you could find a good stretch of ground.

Breakfast: You eat this as late as possible or just have a bigger-than-usual, early lunch, choosing scrambled egg, bacon and asparagus – or maybe an omelet and veg.

Lunch: Organic prawn salad with loads of veggies. Chop up extra vegetables and throw them into a slow cooker; add lots of lamb and cook on slow, ready for tonight's supper.

Supper: Lamb casserole, with some fruit for 'sweet'. You make sure you eat until you're full. *Don't forget the italicised details above.*

(Tonight, after your fasted exercise and then the two good meals, your metabolism is at racing speed. Ideal for fat burning)

THURSDAY:

Breakfast: You eat a light breakfast of nuts, fruits and seeds with a little cream.

Lunch: Steamed fish (wild salmon maybe) and 2 or 3 veg (also steamed.)

You think of something fun to do today: play a friendly game of tennis or squash; or have a kick-around in a park with your kids. You're sure to take it easy though.

Supper: Stuffed butternut squash with mince or a huge rack of ribs (with plenty left over for tomorrow's lunch), adding 2 vegetables of your choice. Take blueberries and a little cream for 'sweet', or a piece of fruit.

Doesn't sound so bad, does it?

Natural lifestyle

Motivation and attitude

It's important to approach this new healthier way of living with some lightness of attitude. To start with, be kind to yourself. You weren't perfect before, and you're not likely to be perfect now. But you are going to do considerably better for yourself, and for your family too if they join you on this challenge. Remember that *any* change is initially tricky but this is a huge opportunity to gain something very special, not just another way to feel bad about yourself when you slip up. It's a journey, an adventure. It *should* be challenging, but also fun.

Get adequate rest and sleep. Go on – go to bed earlier than you do currently. Stop pushing through that late evening slump, accept you're tired and embrace it. Take some time to read or write before you turn the light out.

Give the full eight hours sleep a try for a couple of weeks and see how it impacts on your life. Look carefully at how your evening *usually* pans out, and create a plan to get you to bed by 10 O'clock (preferably

9.00pm) without fail. Set your alarm early enough to enjoy some gentle exercise before you'd normally wake.

Exposure to sunshine and outdoor life. Get out of the concrete jungle from time to time; visit a park or, even better, get out into the country-side and get mucky. Find at least half an hour a day to just get outside and soak up some sunshine. Go for a walk at lunchtime, walk the dog or even just sit in the garden.

Set some time aside each day to walk in the elements. Commit to going whether the sun is shining, the wind is blowing or it's raining and snowy. Make your mind up to celebrate and enjoy the weather in all its glories – get outside for half an hour a day. Stick to it for two weeks and see how you feel.

As Ranulph Fiennes, the world's greatest living explorer once re-marked: "There's no such thing as bad weather, just inappropriate clothing".

Physical challenge and meaningful risk. Look for a range of ways to inject fun, competition or challenge into your physical activities. Strive to make movement part of an everyday task that needs to be completed anyway. If you can't find a meaningful task then make one up: perhaps add a social aspect, make a bet with a friend or colleague, concoct a game or dream up a self-imposed forfeit? The point being that you don't find yourself focused on counting down the minutes and seconds of self-inflicted torture. Remove your mind from the labour and place it firmly on a purpose – any purpose. Instinctive movement is not about striving for fitness goals, it's about moving and enjoying the moment for what it is. Don't worry so much about reps, duration and performance. Find or create great reasons to move your body in an instinctive way. Find a va-riety of excuses for movements that you enjoy, that you find fun – and all your fitness goals will arrive with ease and without further invitation.

Play and festivity. Life shouldn't be a grind – really it shouldn't! More and more we are being told we must work harder and longer to get the economy going. From where I'm standing unless you're the Chancellor of the Exchequer, it isn't your responsibility to do anything other than provide the best life possible for you and your loved ones.

Take some time out from all the work, exercise and preparing food to do something totally for the sheer hell of it. Dance, sing, paint, and enjoy the company of others.

Other consumables. Stand guard at the gate of your own experience. Choose carefully where you place your attention: the television you watch, the papers you read, the people you talk with and the topics you choose to discuss. You really can build up or knock down the world you live in simply by being more discerning about where you spend your time and pay your attention.

Avoid the news for a couple of weeks. The world really will continue to turn without you knowing all its horrors intimately. Let News stories come and go without allowing them polluting *your* life. Observe how the weight of the world's problems melts away when you refuse to be sucked into all the media-driven negativity.

Love and belonging. Rejoice at being part of a family and community. Yes, other people can be a complete pain from time to time, but in the end – we wouldn't be without them. Reach out to the people closest to you and show them that you care in whatever way feels right to you.

Think of that person you care about and have been meaning to call for months. Grab their number, pick up the phone and give them a ring *right now!* No, don't put it off, or 'cop out' by texting or 'FaceBooking'. Speak to them direct, and even better, arrange to meet in person. You'll be glad you did.

It's OK not to be perfect

Please don't aim for anything less than 100%, but it's OK to allow yourself to score as low as 80% some days, or some weeks and still accept your efforts. You will still gain most of the promised benefits if you get things 80% right. (This is sometimes known as the '80/20 rule'.) You can't mess things up very much with one or two bad meals a week or a few days of sedentary living. It's the larger patterns that matter. How many days of good exercise did you fit in this month? How many non-processed meals did you manage to consume this month? This is the scale on which you can start to see the clear results of your efforts.

You're going to make mistakes, have moments of weakness and wander from the path. But it's not the end of the world – seriously. Don't be too tough on yourself. When you go wrong, you go wrong – all that matters is you get back on track.

Please remember that this isn't the promise of a quick-fix, or a short-cut to anything. Ultimately, there are no short-cuts to anything, no matter what the adverts tell you. Short-cuts in health terms are bad and tend to only give the *illusion* of progress. If you want to lose 21 pounds this month, it's easy. Just eat cabbage soup and nothing else. You'll destroy your metabolism, compromise your immune system and likely as not become quite ill – but you *will* have lost those 21 pounds. However if you want sustainable low-fat levels and high levels of health for the rest of your life – well that's different.

Forget unrealistic targets for this week, this month or perhaps even this year. Take a long-term, tortoise-never-the-hare approach – and blow your mind with what you can achieve. Nothing else is congruent with the bodies and genetics we have all been given.

'Instinctive' fitness is based on principles and knowledge of our ancient past. Let your instincts once again work for you – don't be enslaved to them.

That's the key to it really: remember the WHY. Remember why you're doing this.

Picture yourself how you wish you were, and imagine the way you'll feel in a month, a year, even ten years' time if you stick with, and trust in the process. Everything is created twice; once in the mind and only then in reality. What pictures do you have to recreate and when are you going to get started?

If you don't get the results you're hoping for fast enough, ask yourself the following:

- **Am I expecting too much too soon**? *Is it realistic to expect to lose all the fat around your belly while you still have plenty on your arms, for example? This programme isn't a magic bullet for overnight transformation. It is, however, the only programme I know that people can stick with and that will continue to pay dividends for years. You will overtake your friends on their yo-yo diets, not because this programme works faster (it might not do), but because it will keep giving when they have long since quit. It will also be much healthier than their approach.*

- **Am I actually following the principles properly?** *How similar are most of your days to the four example days described above? Or have you got lots of little rationalised cheats going in your mind: "Well potatoes are vegetables aren't they, and if I fry them in coconut oil…"*

241

- **Am I expecting linear improvements?** *Life tends not to work like this. Nobody loses exactly two pounds a week for five months. Your body is much too complicated to be able to affect in such a predictable manner. Some of my clients have lost no weight at all for the first few weeks. Before that though, many started enjoying superior levels of energy and lost two or three inches of grain-bloating around the waist.*

One thing you can do to help your progress is to journalise it. You could do this in a diary next to your bed, or start a blog to update supportive friends. One reason to do this is that it's human nature to forget quickly how much we've achieved and from where we started out. Write down all your basic measurements and some performance benchmarks (press-ups, pull-ups, and squats – that kind of thing.)

These things are not the reasons for eating and living a more natural lifestyle, but they do tend to keep us on track. Another powerful Jedi mind trick is to tell as many people as you're comfortable with about your intention to make a change. We tend to strive subconsciously to live up to the expectations of others, so let this fact work for you. Allow your desire to appear capable and consistent in the eyes of others create a momentum that helps you follow through on your goals.

Having said that, there will be some who will fear you are gaining something that they haven't got the self-discipline or the know-how for, so don't be surprised when someone close to you tries to undermine your efforts. Expect a few of the brainwashed, low-fat crowd to scoff if you disclose an affection for bacon, butter or full-fat, organic cream.

Let your results speak for themselves

When you reach mile stones (e.g. one month without grain), why not reward yourself with a something special to reinforce your achievement? (No, not a large Domino's Pizza)

It's really important that, without departing from any crucial principles, you find ways to enjoy the process of turning things around. Find things that work for you: easy and delicious meals, enjoyable exercises, fun games and sports – that kind of thing. Personalise the programme as much as you can, focusing on the process and not just results.

Banish any images of what you should look like from your mind. Ignore the siren-call of the media for enormous muscles or a wispy, waif-like figure; that's not always written on the genetic cards we were handed at birth. You can still look great with a bigger than average frame if you're female, or with the lean musculature of a Thai-fighter if you're a smaller than average guy. Sometimes learning to feel good about yourself is of greater importance than any possible aesthetic result you might achieve.

Remember also how much more there is to this than a concern with aesthetics. What about living longer? What about staying mobile into your 90s? What about attaining super-charged levels of energy? What about beautiful poise and a pain-free body? This is the meat and bones of true Instinctive Fitness.

This book has not meant to lecture or impose an opinion on you; instead it was intended to offer you a completely new version of the truth. Instinctive Fitness is about making subtle as well as broad changes that will bring you closer in-line with the instincts nature gave you. Every change you make realigns you with the drives that worked so well for our forefathers, the only species of Hominid to survive the ruthless race of evolution.

Here again are those instincts we met at the start of the book and what we can do with each to re-sculpture our bodies and re-launch our lives anew:

Working with your instincts

Put on weight whenever possible: *If you eat the Instinctive Fitness way, eating a high-fat, medium protein, low-carb diet, you'll find putting on weight will actually be difficult. If you start skipping meals for the sake of convenience, it's possible that you may have to guard against being too thin, just like our ancient ancestors did. However, with plenty of protein in your diet and some explosive movement, new weight will come in the form of muscle, rather than fat. Additional muscle burns fat through the day and is one of your best defences against frailty and ill health through-out life. Also, well-toned men and women are more attractive and more capable in every way.*

Crave sweet, salty and fatty foods: *Retrain your taste buds by eating the foods our instincts evolved to direct us towards. Fulfill your appetite for these tastes through a naturally higher-fat diet based around meat, fish, fowl, fruit, seeds, nuts and veg. Re-sensitise yourself to the subtler tastes of good, natural food. When your palate recovers and your brain forgets about the hyper-stimulation it once received from shiny, packeted 'bait' foods and other food imposters, you will lose your cravings and ad-*

dictions, you'll lose fat, and your blood glucose levels will stabilise, providing you with on-tap energy throughout the whole day.

Rest whenever possible: *Build physical tasks into your day so that it's impossible to rest all day long. Ensure you include some explosive movement, maybe using a simple, brief workout routine similar to the one I outlined earlier in the book. Find active things to do that you enjoy doing and turn them into a habit. Learn to play and have fun with movement as you used to as a child. Do ensure that you include plenty of rest, however; avoid excess stress and refrain from overly intensive cardio routines.*

Eat whatever's available and tastes good*: Buy only pure, natural foods; not foods that have been messed about with in factories and have undergone heavy processing. If the supermarket is filled with temptations for you, avoid it, shop elsewhere or shop online. Clear your cupboards of all the junk. Once you're surrounded by real food, you can feel free to eat until you're full and have a really good feast whenever you feel like it. Because your body knows that it is always well provided for, it won't feel the need to store those calories as fat.*

Eat whatever looks shiny, bright and healthy: *Learn to see the product itself. Don't be fooled by shiny packaging and the efforts of the media and advertising to hook your interest. Learn to read ingredients labels, particularly looking out for those danger ingredients: vegetable oil, sugar, sweeteners, etc. Ask yourself, is this food part of a natural eco-chain, or is it just 'bait' laid out to trap my well-meaning instinct?*

Wake up when it's light and sleep when it's dark: *Go to bed when you first start to get tired between 9-10pm. Sleep with the curtains open and wake up slowly and naturally as the morning light streams into your bedroom. Avoid excessive time spent in front of a screen as this will affect your ability to sleep deeply and wake rested.*

Copy the posture and movement of these around us*: Look out for better role models – like some athletes and many non-westerners who still move with the grace and poise that we all should.*

Finally, once you've found your feet, don't forget your duty to spread the word. For too long we've been at the mercy of bad advice from government health advisors, from an ignorant media and from scientists stuck in dogmatic cul-de-sacs.

In evolutionary and genetic terms we are perfect; in environmental and behavioural terms we have seriously handicapped ourselves. Only when enough people are willing to think for themselves and kick against the boards will the balance tip. Then we can create a new generation of people who are free to enjoy all the blessings that form our inheritance – if we only had the instinct and the wisdom to see it.

That's it then; all you need. However some readers will prefer reading about this than actually taking action. I am always frustrated by people who find excuses and fail to take the first step to turn their lives around. Those that do, usually say one of a few things.

'Sorry excuses' often trotted out...

1. "I don't have time"

You don't have enough time on the planet *not* to make these changes. Everybody has the same amount of time in the day as the next person; what they lack is priority. If they choose not to implement these changes, then fine – but be honest and say "It's not that important to me". The approach I've outlined here is based on the 'minimal effective dose' idea: how to get the most out of the smallest investment in your time.

2. "I don't have the money"

Much of what's in this programme is free. You don't need a gym subscription. You don't need to buy any equipment unless you choose to. You don't need special supplements. You will be saving money on gym memberships, medical bills and overpriced, starch-filled 'peasant food' with no nutritional value. I will concede that your meat and vegetable bill might go up but, having said that, I can't think of a more important thing to invest in than your future health and happiness. 'Health is wealth,' as the saying goes. Of the many areas in your life where you can save money, why choose your own wellbeing?

3. "I haven't got the self-discipline and it seems a bit complicated."

To me it seems simple, but it's part of my nature now; habit has made it easy. I agree, though, that any change can be difficult in the early days. I would encourage you to get help if you can. If you're organized, you can make the changes and feel benefits pretty quickly, so ask for support from a personal trainer, a partner, friends – anybody who understands fully what you're up to. With my own clients I organise everything for them – the weekly food ordering, the weekly meal plan, and the daily exercise – so that it's as easy as it possibly can be. I've organised my free 30-day IF Programme in just the same way, showing people how they can make the transition in small, comfortable steps. Just sign-up on the website: www.instinctive-fitness.com

4. "I'm not convinced it will work. What if it doesn't?"

Well what will you have you lost? Now compare this loss with the almost guaranteed loss of health and mobility that you face if you do nothing. Make your best choice and act now. The only way to know is to try. Every few hours that passes after you put this book down means that you're more likely to fall back into the habits that have got you to where you are now.

5. "I'll do this – it *does* make sense. Just not now. Next month will be better when..."

Most people believe they should wait for conditions to be right before they act. This attitude doesn't work. Ever. The one that does is "Do what you can, now" The conditions will never be perfect, no matter how long you wait. If you can't face taking action right now, at least commit to learn more, read more; find out the truth behind the issues this book has presented.

Don't lose momentum – do something right now

Hopefully you'll now leap up, head outside out and start moving, or pop across to www.instinctive-fitness.com for our 30-Day Eating Challenge. But perhaps you're one of those people who always demand yet more convincing? Knowledge is never a bad thing so you might like to head down your local bookshop for some further reading. Below you'll find some of the pivotal books that helped inspire our Instinctive Eating approach:

The Primal Blueprint by Mark Sisson

Discover more about the cold, hard nutritional science with Mark Sisson, perhaps someone who has done more to popularise the Paleo movement than any other with this standout book and fantastic blog. Not necessarily the easiest read as it digs right down into the detail of human anatomy and physiology, but if you want to really understand the minutiae of how your body works then we think this will be right up your ally.

Stop Counting Calories & Start Losing Weight by Zoë Harcombe

For those people specifically looking to lose weight this book will explain you why you cannot help but overeat due to the three commonly overlooked medical conditions which can cause insatiable food cravings. It offers you a way to overcome these three conditions and to end food addiction and overeating.

Zoë clearly explains how we all essentially eat emotionally, and how early childhood messages impact us. A book not driven by our ancestral past but all the same we feel makes a superlative case against the misguided mainstream wisdom of low fat, high carb diets.

The Paleo Diet Cookbook by Dr. Loren Cordain

Dr. Loren is a research scientist who must be credited as one of the key founders of the ancestral health movement. This is simply a great cookbook from one of the original inspirations behind the Instinctive Eating philosophy, showing how the diet of our Paleolithic ancestors can be brought into the 21st century. It offers more than 150 satisfying recipes packed with great flavours and enough variety to help you enjoy all the benefits of eating the Paleo way.

Everyday Paleo, by Sarah Fragoso

Another book we highly recommend because it offers detailed instructions for acquiring and maintaining a Paleo lifestyle to improve the health and longevity of your whole family. Sarah Fragoso shows how living naturally is a whole lifestyle, not just another fad diet. It's a great mum's perspective on how to get your whole family on board with this new way of doing things.

Trick and Treat by Barry Groves

This is another favourite book. Barry shows how the British health industry is ruled by the multinational pharmaceutical and big food companies. It is they who really control what health professionals are taught and make doctors, nutritionists and dieticians into unwitting mouthpieces and drug pushers. Trick and Treat shows that there is, however, a way out. While the 'health industry' tries to make everyone into 'patients', we don't have to comply, and we don't have to get ill. Live the right lifestyle and they cannot force us to take their drugs and unnatural 'foods' if we don't want to. We love it.

The Paleo Solution by Robb Wolf

A scientist and powerlifter, Robb Wolf explains how if you can lose fat and stay young, all while avoiding cancer, diabetes, heart disease, Parkinson's, Alzheimer's and a host of other illnesses. The Paleo Solution incorporates the latest, cutting edge research from genetics, biochemistry and anthropology to help you look, feel and perform your best. Well worth reading.

Time to get your body moving...

By now you should understand how you really don't need a fancy gym membership to start moving your body more. You don't need any money, equipment, a club, a class or even any indoor space. As was explained in the Movement Chapter, you really can get your body moving again by doing absolutely anything that involves more effort than stretching an arm across to the TV remote control.

Having said all that, there are some fantastic organisations out there who can offer some form and structure to your new enthusiasm to get in shape.

MovNat

MovNat (which stands for Move Naturally) has been mentioned a couple of times in this book already – and for good reason. Their purity of philosophy, delivery and the inspiration they offer anyone looking for genuine 'real world' fitness is exemplary.

I asked Master MovNat instructor, Vic Verdier, who kindly wrote the foreword to this book to describe MovNat in a nut shell. In his own words:

MovNat is a physical education & fitness system based on training the full range of our natural human movement abilities. MovNat is safe, progressive and fully scaleable. Erwan Le Corre, MovNat's founder, wants everyone to 'explore their true nature' – a right to live a long, healthy, physically active and happy life. MovNat training activities include running, balancing, walking, crawling, jumping, climbing, swimming, grappling, striking, lifting, carrying, throwing and catching. MovNat can be practiced everywhere – a park, beach, forest or in a city. MovNat's mission it is to revolutionise current thinking around fitness and physical education with a return to real-world physical competency, health and well-being.

MovNat's no-compromise approach to the purest forms of human movement serves as both a model to follow and a source of inspiration for a growing number of people dissatisfied with automated exercise. It's perfect for those who want to return to their ancestral roots to once again enjoy exercise and celebrate their physicality.

A picture tells a thousand words, and a good video clip tells a whole lot more – so tap 'MovNat' into YouTube, sit back and enjoy the ride.

Oh, you're back already? Inspiring stuff, isn't it? You might already be thinking of trees to climb or rock faces to scale. For me at least, it's the ultimate expression of using your body how nature intended it to be used. You can get even more inspired at www.movnat.com.

It's not for everyone though: you might be thinking that MovNat isn't perhaps the best route for you to personally start reclaiming your fitness. To be honest for some people it's a little 'far out there' to even begin emulating the antics of Erwan or Vic on a daily basis. Luckily there are other options:

Crossfit

Also mentioned earlier in the book, we consider CrossFit to be the more accessible 'urban' face of functional fitness. Founded by Greg Glassman in 2000, CrossFit's exercise programs are now practiced by members of approximately 4,400 affiliated gyms, most of which are located in the United States. The CrossFit ethos has now spread around the world with (at the time of writing) around 80 gyms up and running here in the UK.

Unlike most impersonal, homogenised conventional gyms, CrossFit offers a genuine everyday opportunity for anyone to build an almost unparalleled level of all round fitness and agility within easy reach of most urban centres. Another aspect we particularly like about the CrossFit culture is they nurture a much friendlier, welcoming and more inclusive feel to their membership; so if you want your gym to have eye-wateringly expensive 'energy drink' machines in every room, polished lockers and a walnut reception desk – best look elsewhere. If you simply want to get in serious shape, happen to have a CrossFit gym local to you and enjoy a feeling of purpose and team spirit, www.crossfit.com may well be worth a look.

Woodland Workouts

Closer to home, the Instinctive Fitness Team offers everyday people the opportunity to get involved in the more practical side of our movement philosophy through our various Woodland Workout groups.

Steadily growing in the North Oxfordshire area of England, we have put together a range of structured but fun sessions to get individuals at all levels of fitness moving again within England's beautiful natural environment. No matter what your physical condition right now, we offer a really accessible opportunity to get back in touch with your ancestral roots and once again move your body the way it was designed to move.

Woodland Workouts are about reenergizing both body and soul without the blood, sweat and tears associated with traditional boot-camp-style workouts; so if painless exercise with a light touch and an attitude of utter playfulness is your thing, perhaps take a look at: www.woodland-workouts.co.uk

The Gokhale Method

85-90% of the western world population has at some point in their life suffered from a foot, knee, hip and back problem (a truly astonishing number). The chances are then that you've been there too. If so, it might be worth looking into what the real underlying causes are.

Esther Gokhale discovered the answer when travelling and researching postural related pain in areas of Africa, India, Brazil and Southern Europe where, despite many hours of both sedentary and active work, only around 5% of adults reported any experience of back pain.

Preserved in the kinaesthetic traditions of these peoples, Gokhale observed a common body-wisdom from which she formed the blueprint for the Gokhale Method. This highly successful program of postural re-education has been developed and successfully taught at the Gokhale Institute in Palo Alto, California over the past 20 years.

In her widely acclaimed 2008 book, '8 Steps to a Pain-Free Back', Gokhale made her revolutionary findings available to the general public with practical support from teachers in the States, the UK, Europe and India. If you're sick of popping painkillers to get through your day, then perhaps bad posture is the real underlying problem? If you'd like to find out where your nearest Gokhale Method teacher is and how they can help you go to: www.gokhalemethod.com

Parkour or Free Running

This is a great option for those hemmed in by the city on all sides. Parkour is the physical discipline of travelling through challenging urban environments with the greatest amount of efficiency, grace and joi-de-vivre. Learn to master the urban jungle with movements that could make you resemble Tarzan in a tracksuit. Leaping, vaulting, jumping, rolling, swinging, crawling and climbing are all on the curriculum. Much safer than you would think, it is taught brilliantly, passionately and in an inspired fashion all over London by Parkour Generations. It's genuinely for people of all ages and backgrounds. You certainly don't need a hoodie and teenage angst to train! For more information, see www.parkourgenerations.com

Bring on the challenge

You've now surfed the web, read the books and perhaps even got the T-Shirt, but there does come a point when research and thoroughness of preparation turns into goal-jeopardising procrastination.

Once you've got sufficient information then no more excuses – it's time for action. If you're ready to start planning and taking those vital first steps without further ado, you might like to download our 30-Day Challenge from www.instinctive-fitness.com and see how easy it really is to start turning your health around.

A new age with new hope

The world really is slowly waking up to a more natural way of eating, exercising and living, however this isn't the time for any of us to get complacent, self-congratulate and sit back and relax. To reclaim the nations health we all need to do our bit to harness and combine our voices to make them louder than the corrosive, self-serving but incredibly well-funded corporate message of what still passes for consumer health advice. Every extra whisper of truth helps our planet become happier, healthier and live longer, and a global army of whispers makes a lot of noise – so start whispering.

Changing any accepted world view is always going to be an uphill battle – and it's especially hard when a blatantly erroneous (but profitable) version of truth is perpetuated by the institutions that power world politics and a global economy. If you are convinced by the facts we've presented – facts you might have initially thought 'way out', then please help spread the word.

Tell your friends and family; buy them a book, perhaps write a review on Amazon; post a few words on your blog or Facebook page, or use whatever other means you may have to reach out to the people who don't yet know and who really matter.

On a more personal note, we also love to hear how Instinctive Fitness has changed your life so we can keep up the pressure and spread the word on your behalf. Stories of both challenge and success are welcomed, so please let us know how this book has changed things for you via email to personalrevolution@instinctive-fitness.com.

A final thought

So as you ponder over these last few words, you might still be questioning whether everything you've just read here is true and wonder whether it will it really make a huge difference to your life? After all, perhaps it somehow won't work for you or you might fall short of perfection as you may have done in the past?

Worrying, wondering and fretting about what's gone before and what might follow won't change the decision you must make right now in this moment. Are you going to carry on as you have been or are you ready to grab your future with both hands and regain control of the animal instincts that served your ancestors so well? Go on...

Choose to once more eat like a king, play like a child and live your life to the full. Take a leap of faith, return to your instincts, look forward to the past and unleash your fitter, stronger and happier caveman within.

"Men occasionally stumble over the truth, but most of them pick themselves up and hurry off as if nothing ever happened."
Sir Winston Churchill

References:

1. Daniel E. Lieberman et al. (2010) "Foot strike patterns and collision forces in habitually barefoot versus shod runners." Nature 463, 531-535

About the Authors

Born in 1975, Oliver Selway lives in Oxford, UK. Besides being a writer, Oliver is, as the Sunday Times described him, a 'radical diet and fitness coach'. He gave up his job in journalism to retrain and change people's lives after transforming his own body and health with a system that confounds the advice of conventional trainers and gyms. He wrote *Instinctive Fitness* to let people struggling to stay slim, healthy and energetic know that there is a better way than stress, striving and usually failing.

Charlie Packer, born in 1970, is a collaborative writer who works with people with important things to say – but don't quite know how to say them. Medically retired after 14 years as a fire-fighter with worn out knees, Charlie began struggling with fitness and weight issues. A fortuitous meeting with Olly led to a new diet, a new exercise programme and ultimately a new book. Losing nearly 2 stone in weight and nearly all his knee pain in less than 4 months, Charlie knows first-hand how well the Instinctive Fitness approach works.

We'd love to hear about your experiences, so please do get in touch through the website or find us on Facebook.

www.instinctive-fitness.com
info@instinctive-fitness.com

Bibliography

Academic

The Descent of Man by Charles Darwin and Michael T. Ghiselin *(Jan 14, 2010)*

Man the Hunter by Irven Devore and Richard B. Lee *(Dec 31, 1999)*

Limited Wants, Unlimited Means: A Reader on Hunter-Gatherer Economics and The Environment by John Gowdy *(Dec 1, 1997)*

First Farmers: The Origins of Agricultural Societies by Peter S. Bellwood *(Dec 6, 2004)*

Catching Fire: How Cooking Made Us Human by Richard W. Wrangham *(Sep 7, 2010)*

Evolution and Prehistory: The Human Challenge by William A. Haviland, etc. *(Mar 5, 2010)*

The Lost World of the Kalahari by Laurens Van Der Post *(Nov 3, 1977)*

Primitive Man & His Food by Arnold De Vries *(1900)*

Myth and Meaning: Cracking the Code of Culture by Claude Levi-Strauss *(Mar 14, 1995)*

Guns, Germs, and Steel: The Fates of Human Societies by Jared Diamond *(Jul 11, 2005)*

Lucy's Child: the Discovery of a Human Ancestor by Donald C. Johanson *(Oct 31, 1991)*

The World of Primitive Man by Paul Radin and Stanley Diamond *(1971 (Nov 9, 2007)*

Against Civilization: Readings and Reflections by John Zerzan *(May 10, 2005)*

Food and Western Disease: Health and nutrition from an evolutionary perspective by Staffan Lindeberg (January 19, 2010)

The Omnivore's Dilemma: A Natural History of Four Meals by Michael Pollan *(Aug 28, 2007)*

Popular science

The Primal Blueprint: Reprogram your genes for effortless weight loss, vibrant health, and boundless energy by Mark Sisson *(Jan 14, 2012)*

The Paleo Answer: 7 Days to Lose Weight, Feel Great, Stay Young by Loren Cordain *(Dec 20, 2011)*

The New Evolution Diet: What Our Paleolithic Ancestors Can Teach Us about Weight Loss, Fitness, and Aging by Arthur De Vany and Nassim Nicholas Taleb *(Dec 20, 2011)*

The Obesity Epidemic: What caused it? How can we stop it? By Zoë Harcombe (Oct 2010)

8 Steps to a Pain-Free Back: Natural Posture Solutions for Pain in the Back, Neck, Shoulder, Hip, Knee, and Foot by Esther Gokhale and Susan Adams *(Apr 1, 2008)*

The Paleo Solution: The Original Human Diet by Robb Wolf and Loren Cordain Ph.D. *(Sep 14, 2010)*

Food Inc.: How Industrial Food is Making Us Sicker, Fatter, and Poorer-And What You Can Do About It by Participant Media and Karl Weber *(May 5, 2009)*

Good Calories, Bad Calories: Fats, Carbs, and the Controversial Science of Diet and Health by Gary Taubes *(23 Sep 2008)*

The Great Cholesterol Con by Dr. Malcolm Kendrick *(7 Jul 2008)*

Wheat Belly: Lose the Wheat, Lose the Weight, and Find Your Path Back to Health by William Davis *(Aug 30, 2011)*

Beyond Broccoli: Creating a Biologically Balanced Diet When a Vegetarian Diet Doesn't Work by Susan Schenck Lac and Bob Avery *(Aug 20, 2011)*

Nourishing Traditions: the Cookbook that Challenges Politically Correct Nutrition and the Diet Dictocrats by Sally Fallon (1st September 2009)

Websites

http://www.marksdailyapple.com/ (Mark Sisson, #1 Paleo blogger)

http://www.thepaleodiet.com (Loren Cordain, esteemed scientist and early proponent of Paleo)

http://www.proteinpower.com/drmike/ (blog of Micheal Eades, MD)

http://vimeo.com/ancestralhealthsymposium/videos (a meeting of Paleo minds)

http://egwellness.com/what-hurts/lower-back-pain (Esther Gokhale's approach to natural posture)

http://www.posetech.com/ (find your perfect running style)

http://www.bigbarn.co.uk (find local food)

http://www.westonaprice.org/ (Weston A. Price Foundation)

http://barefootrunning.fas.harvard.edu (barefoot running with Daniel Lieberman)

http://www.anatomyinmotion.co.uk (Gary Ward, UK #1 human movement expert for unsolvable pain)

http://www.movnat.com (natural movement with Erwan Le Corre)

http://www.paleohacks.com (ask any Paleo questions)

http://www.primallifestyle.com (Fivefinger shoes)

INDEX